Victor Djimbila Kazadi

A True Plunge into the Heart of the Human Body 2

Victor Djimbila Kazadi

A True Plunge into the Heart of the Human Body 2

Master Therapeutic and Surgical Excellence

ScienciaScripts

Imprint

Cover image: www.ingimage.com

This book is a translation from the original published under ISBN 978-620-6-71361-6.

Publisher:
Sciencia Scripts
is a trademark of
Dodo Books Indian Ocean Ltd. and OmniScriptum S.R.L publishing group

120 High Road, East Finchley, London, N2 9ED, United Kingdom
Str. Armeneasca 28/1, office 1, Chisinau MD-2012, Republic of Moldova, Europe
Managing Directors: Ieva Konstantinova, Victoria Ursu
info@omniscriptum.com

Printed at: see last page
ISBN: 978-620-8-60310-6

Table of contents

Foreword

In an ever-changing world, where technological advances and scientific discoveries are constantly redefining the healthcare landscape, it is imperative for healthcare professionals to acquire a specialization that goes beyond theoretical knowledge. This book takes an in-depth look at innovative therapies, modern surgical techniques and therapeutic communication methods, with an emphasis on the "learning-by-doing" pedagogical approach.

The "Learnig-by-doing" method is based on the idea that learning is optimized when individuals are actively engaged in their educational process. By integrating this approach into the training of healthcare professionals, we promote not only a better understanding of complex concepts, but also the development of essential practical skills. This enables practitioners to apply their knowledge directly to real-life clinical situations, boosting their confidence and efficiency.

Innovative therapies represent a dynamic field that requires continuous updating of skills. New therapeutic approaches, whether pharmacological or based on non-invasive interventions, require a thorough understanding of the underlying mechanisms, as well as the ability to evaluate their efficacy in a variety of clinical settings. Similarly, modern surgical techniques are evolving rapidly with the introduction of technologies such as robotics and computer-assisted surgery. These innovations require not only rigorous technical training, but also the ability to communicate effectively with patients and multidisciplinary teams.

Therapeutic communication is another fundamental aspect that deserves particular attention. The way a professional interacts with his or her patients can have a significant impact on the healing process. Clear, empathetic communication not only promotes adherence to treatment, but also helps establish a relationship of trust between patient and practitioner.

Veritable Plongée au Coeur du Corps Humain" aims to provide readers not only with theoretical knowledge, but also with the practical tools to excel in these crucial areas. Through case studies, practical exercises and expert testimonials, we hope to inspire a new generation of professionals to integrate these skills into their daily practice.

In conclusion, as we embark on this in-depth exploration of innovative therapies, modern surgical techniques and effective therapeutic communication strategies, we invite every reader to adopt a proactive attitude towards their learning. The future of healthcare will largely depend on our collective ability to innovate and adapt our practices to the changing needs of our patients.

Victor Djimbila Kazadi: Our Father

MODULE 1: INNOVATIVE THERAPY

Chapter 1: Molecular and cellular biology

In-depth, hands-on studies in molecular and cell biology encompass a wide range of techniques, concepts and applications that are essential for understanding the fundamental mechanisms of life at the molecular level. Molecular biology focuses on the interactions between different biological systems, in particular the interactions between DNA, RNA and proteins. Cell biology, on the other hand, examines the structure and function of cells, including their organelles and communication.

Fundamental concepts

- **DNA and RNA**: Deoxyribonucleic acid (DNA) is the genetic material that carries the information necessary for the reproduction and functioning of living organisms. Ribonucleic acid (RNA) plays a crucial role in protein synthesis, acting as an intermediary between DNA and ribosomes.

- **Protein synthesis**: This process comprises several key steps: transcription (where DNA is copied into messenger RNA) and translation (where messenger RNA is used to assemble amino acids into proteins).

- **Molecular Biology techniques**: Commonly used techniques include PCR (polymerase chain reaction), DNA sequencing, gene cloning, as well as gene manipulation methods such as CRISPR-Cas9.

- **Cell culture**: Cell culture is used to study the behavior of cells in a controlled environment. This includes cell growth, differentiation and responses to external stimuli.

- **Practical applications**: The knowledge gained from these studies has a wide range of applications in the medical field (gene therapy), in agriculture (GMOs), and in fundamental research to better understand diseases.

Educational importance

Molecular and cellular biology study programs are often designed to provide hands-on training for students so that they can gain direct experience with these advanced techniques. This involves not only theoretical understanding but also practical competence in the laboratory.

I. Basic molecular biology techniques

a) **DNA and RNA extraction**: The first step in many molecular biology techniques is to isolate DNA or RNA from a biological sample. This may involve chemical or physical methods to lyse cells and purify nucleic acids.

b) **PCR (Polymerase Chain Reaction) amplification**: This technique specifically amplifies a DNA sequence. Using specific primers, PCR produces millions of copies of a targeted region of DNA, facilitating analysis.

c) **Sequencing**: DNA sequencing is crucial for determining the exact sequence of nucleotide bases in a DNA fragment. Modern methods include Sanger sequencing and next-generation sequencing, which enable the genome to be analyzed quickly and efficiently.

d) **Cloning**: Molecular cloning involves the insertion of a DNA fragment into a vector (such as a plasmid) that can be introduced into a host cell to produce multiple copies of the inserted fragment. This is essential for the production of recombinant proteins or for studying genes in detail.

e) **Electrophoretic analysis**: Gel electrophoresis is used to separate nucleic acids or proteins according to size and electrical charge. This technique is often used after PCR or cloning to check the presence and size of amplified or cloned products.

f) **Hybridization**: Hybridization techniques, such as Northern blotting (for RNA) or Southern blotting (for DNA), enable the detection of specific sequences within a complex mixture, using labeled probes that bind to complementary targets.

g) **CRISPR-Cas9**: A revolutionary technique enabling precise genome editing by specifically targeting a DNA sequence to introduce modifications, whether by insertion, deletion or replacement.

h) **Proteomic analysis**: Although mainly focused on nucleic acids, molecular biology also includes the study of proteins via various techniques such as chromatography, mass spectrometry and Western blots.

These interconnected techniques enable researchers not only to explore the molecular basis of various biological processes, but also to apply this knowledge to diverse fields such as medical diagnostics, therapeutic development and even sustainable agriculture.

A. Amplification by PCR (Polymerance Chain Reaction)

PCR (Polymerase Chain Reaction) amplification is a fundamental technique in molecular biology, enabling the exponential multiplication of specific DNA segments. Developed in the 1980s by Kary Mullis, PCR has revolutionized genetic research, medical diagnosis and criminal analysis, among other fields.

PCR basics: PCR is based on three main steps: denaturation, hybridization and elongation.

- **Denaturation**: The first step involves heating the reaction mixture to around 94-98°C to separate the double-stranded DNA strands into single strands.

- **Hybridization**: The temperature is then lowered to around 50-65°C to enable the primers (short DNA sequences) to bind to complementary regions on the target DNA strands.

- **Elongation**: The temperature is raised to around 72°C, promoting the activity of DNA polymerase, an enzyme that synthesizes a new strand of DNA by adding nucleotides complementary to the primers.

These three steps are generally repeated between 25 and 35 cycles, enabling exponential amplification of the targeted DNA segment.

PCR applications: PCR has a variety of applications:

- **Medical diagnostics**: Used to detect viral or bacterial infections by amplifying specific sequences present in pathogens.
- **Genetic research**: studies specific genes and their variations within populations.
- **Criminal analysis**: Used in forensic investigations to amplify DNA from biological traces at crime scenes.
- **Gene cloning**: Facilitates the creation of clones of a particular gene for functional studies or to produce recombinant proteins.

Innovations and improvements: Since its invention, several variants and improvements of PCR have been developed:

- **Real-time PCR (qPCR)**: Allows precise quantification of amplified DNA in real time using fluorescent dyes.
- **Multiplex PCR**: Allows the simultaneous amplification of several DNA targets in the same reaction tube.
- **Digital PCR**: Offers a more sensitive and precise method for quantifying DNA copies by partitioning the reaction mixture.

B. DNA sequencing

DNA sequencing is a fundamental technique in molecular biology for determining the order of nucleotides in a DNA fragment. This method has revolutionized genetics, biotechnology and medicine, providing crucial information on gene structure and function.

1. History of DNA sequencing

DNA sequencing was first introduced in the 1970s by Frederick Sanger, who developed a method known as the Sanger method or chain-termination sequencing. This technique relies on the use of dideoxynucleotides (ddNTPs) which terminate DNA synthesis when incorporated into a growing strand. The subsequent development of high-throughput sequencing methods has accelerated the process considerably, making it possible to sequence the entire human genome.

2. Modern sequencing methods

Modern techniques include Next Generation Sequencing (NGS), which enables the simultaneous sequencing of millions of DNA extracts. Platforms such as Illumina, Ion Torrent and PacBio use different approaches to read nucleotide bases with high precision and low cost. These technologies have paved the way for diverse applications such as metagenomic sequencing, targeted sequencing and exome sequencing.

3. Sequencing applications: DNA sequencing has a wide range of applications:

- **Biomedical research**: Identifying genetic mutations associated with disease.
- **Personalized medicine**: Adaptation of medical treatments based on an individual's genetic profile.
- **Agriculture**: Crop improvement through marker-assisted selection.
- **Ecology**: Study of biodiversity using the environmental metagenome.

4. Ethical and technical challenges

Despite its advantages, DNA sequencing also raises ethical concerns, particularly with regard to the confidentiality of genetic data and the implications for predictive testing. In addition, technical challenges include the management of the massive data generated by NGS technologies, as well as the biological interpretation of results.

5. Future prospects

The future of DNA sequencing looks promising as new technologies continue to emerge that further improve the speed and accuracy of the process. Innovative approaches such as oxidation-based sequencing or nanometric systems could transform our understanding of the human genome and other organisms.

C. Gene cloning

Gene cloning is a fundamental technique in molecular biology, enabling the creation of identical copies of a gene or DNA sequence. The method has a wide range of applications, from basic research to biotechnology and medicine. In-depth studies on gene cloning cover many aspects, including the techniques used, ethical implications and practical applications.

Gene cloning techniques

The gene cloning process generally begins with the extraction of DNA from a donor organism. This DNA is then digested with restriction enzymes that cut the DNA at specific sites, producing DNA fragments. These fragments can be inserted into a vector - often a plasmid - which is then introduced into a host cell by transformation. Once inside the host cell, the vector replicates with the host DNA, enabling the production of numerous copies of the target gene.

Modern methods also include PCR (polymerase chain reaction) cloning, where specific segments of DNA are amplified before insertion into a vector. Homologous recombination cloning is another advanced technique, enabling precise integration of the gene into the host genome.

Gene cloning applications

The applications of gene cloning are vast and include:

- **Biomedical research**: Gene cloning enables researchers to study gene functions by isolating and analyzing their protein products.
- **Production of therapeutic proteins**: Many proteins used as drugs, such as insulin or monoclonal antibodies, are produced by gene cloning.
- **Genetic engineering**: Gene cloning is essential to create genetically modified organisms (GMOs) that can have improved characteristics for agriculture or research.
- **Gene therapy**: This approach uses cloning to introduce corrective genes into human cells to treat certain genetic diseases.

Ethical considerations

Gene cloning also raises important ethical questions. Concerns include the potential risks associated with GMOs for the environment and human health, as well as the moral implications of human and animal cloning. Debates around informed consent and intellectual property rights over genes are also crucial.

D. Electrophoretic analysis

Electrophoretic analysis is a fundamental technique in molecular biology and biochemistry, used to separate macromolecules such as proteins and nucleic acids according to size, charge and conformation. The method is based on the principle of molecule migration in an electric field through a gel or separation medium. In-depth, practical studies of this technique cover many aspects, including types of electrophoresis, applications, experimental protocols and interpretation of results.

Types of electrophoresis

- **Agarose gel electrophoresis**: Mainly used to separate nucleic acids (DNA and RNA). The agarose gel enables efficient resolution of DNA fragments according to their size.

- **Polyacrylamide gel electrophoresis (PAGE)**: This method is often used for protein separation. PAGE can be performed under denaturing (SDS-PAGE) or non-denaturing conditions, enabling analysis of the native structure of proteins.

- **Capillary electrophoresis**: A modern technique that uses very fine capillaries to separate analytes quickly and efficiently.

Applications : Electrophoresis is widely used in various fields:

- **Genetic analysis**: DNA identification and typing for medical diagnosis and genetic studies.
- **Protein characterization**: Analysis of the protein profile in different biological samples, which is crucial for biomedical research.
- **Quality control**: checking the purity and integrity of biopharmaceutical products.

Experimental protocols: Electrophoresis protocols vary according to the type of gel used and the purpose of the analysis. In general, they include:

- Gel preparation (choose the appropriate percentage according to target size).
- Loading samples into gel wells.
- Application of an electric field to induce migration.
- Gel staining after electrophoresis to visualize separated bands.

Interpretation of results: Interpretation requires a thorough understanding of the physical and chemical characteristics of the molecules analyzed. Results are often visualized as bands on the gel, whose position and intensity can be quantified using specialized software.

E. Hybrid techniques

Hybrid techniques are often used in fields such as engineering, biology, education and the arts, where the fusion of several approaches can lead to significant innovations.

Definition of Hybrid Techniques

Hybrid techniques can be defined as methods that integrate two or more distinct systems or approaches to create a new framework for analysis or practice. For example, in the field of engineering, we can observe the use of hybrid systems that combine mechanical and electronic elements to develop more efficient devices. In education, hybrid teaching methods blend e-learning with face-to-face learning to offer a more enriching learning experience.

Practical Applications

- **Engineering**: Hybrid systems are widely used in robotics, where robots can combine artificial intelligence algorithms with mechanical sensors to navigate their environment. This enables better adaptation to unforeseen changes.

- **Biology**: In biotechnology, hybrid techniques involve combining traditional cell culture methods with modern technologies such as CRISPR to genetically modify organisms.

- **Education**: Hybrid learning has become popular in academic institutions, where it combines the best of online and face-to-face courses. This enables students to access a variety of learning materials while benefiting from direct interaction with their teachers.

- **Arts**: In the arts, artists often use hybrid techniques, combining different media (e.g. painting and sculpture) to create innovative works that defy traditional conventions.

- **Information technology**: Hybrid IT architectures integrate both cloud computing and on-premises infrastructures to optimize data management and improve security.

Importance of Hybrid Technology Research

Research into these techniques is crucial, not only for improving efficiency in various fields, but also for encouraging interdisciplinary innovation. By studying how different approaches can be effectively integrated, researchers can develop new solutions to the complex problems facing our society today.

F. CRISPR-Cas

CRISPR-Cas, an acronym for "Clustered Regularly Interspaced Short Palindromic Repeats" and "CRISPR-associated protein", represents a revolutionary technology in the field of molecular biology and genetics. This method enables genes to be edited with unprecedented precision, opening up promising prospects for biomedical research, agriculture and even gene therapy.

1. Origin and mechanism

The CRISPR-Cas system was discovered in bacteria, where it serves as a defense mechanism against viruses. Bacteria use DNA sequences called CRISPR to store fragments of viral DNA, enabling them to recognize and target these viruses in subsequent infections. The system also includes Cas proteins, such as Cas9, which act like molecular scissors to cut DNA in specific places.

2. Research applications

The applications of CRISPR-Cas are vast. In basic research, it is used to create genetically modified animal models to study human diseases. For example, by targeting specific genes associated with certain pathologies such as cancer or neurodegenerative diseases, researchers can better understand the mechanisms underlying these conditions.

3. Medical applications

In the medical field, CRISPR-Cas offers the possibility of developing gene therapies to correct genetic mutations responsible for hereditary diseases. Clinical trials are already underway to treat conditions such as sickle-cell anemia and certain forms of hereditary blindness.

4. Ethics and Regulation

However, the use of CRISPR also raises important ethical questions. The possibility of editing the human genome raises moral dilemmas concerning hereditary modification and the implications for human evolution. Many countries have introduced strict regulations concerning the use of this technology in research and medicine.

5. Future prospects

As our understanding of the CRISPR-Cas system deepens, it is likely that its applications will continue to expand. Research is underway to improve the specificity of gene targeting in order to minimize off-target effects, which could make this technology even safer and more effective.

II. Gene manipulation and gene therapy

Gene manipulation, which includes techniques such as genome editing, enables scientists to modify an organism's genetic material. This can be achieved by a variety of methods, the best known of which are CRISPR-Cas9, TALENs (Transcription Activator-Like Effector Nucleases) and ZFNs (Zinc Finger Nucleases). These technologies offer unprecedented precision in targeting specific DNA sequences, making it possible to correct mutations responsible for hereditary diseases.

Gene therapy is a clinical application of these techniques. It aims to treat or prevent disease by introducing, deleting or modifying genetic material within a patient's cells. Approaches can include the insertion of healthy genes to replace defective ones, or the direct correction of mutations. The first clinical applications have been successfully realized in the treatment of certain genetic diseases such as adrenoleukodystrophy or certain forms of immunodeficiency.

The ethical and technical challenges associated with these practices are also considerable. Questions surrounding the safety of genetic modification, the implications for future generations and the ethical considerations surrounding human genome editing are at the heart of contemporary debates. In addition, the regulations surrounding these technologies vary considerably between countries, influencing their development and implementation.

III. Biotechnology and drug development

1. Introduction to biotechnology

Biotechnology is defined as the use of biological systems or living organisms to develop or create products. It encompasses a variety of techniques from genetic manipulation to cell culture. Biopharmaceutical applications include the production of monoclonal antibodies, vaccines and other therapeutic agents.

2. **New drug development**

- **Genomics and proteomics:** Genomics involves the study of an organism's genome, enabling researchers to identify genes associated with specific diseases. Proteomics, on the other hand, focuses on the study of the proteins expressed by these genes. Together, these disciplines provide an in-depth understanding of the molecular mechanisms underlying human disease.
- **Screening techniques:** High-throughput screening techniques are essential to the drug discovery process. They make it possible to rapidly assess the biological activity of a large number of chemical compounds on specific targets. This considerably speeds up the traditional process, which was previously long and costly.
- **Bioproduction:** Biotechnology is also used to produce complex biomolecules such as monoclonal antibodies and vaccines. These biological products are often more effective and have fewer side effects than traditional synthetic drugs.
- **Gene and cell therapy:** advances in gene therapy offer the possibility of treating certain hereditary diseases by correcting or replacing defective genes. Similarly, cell therapy uses stem cells to regenerate or repair damaged tissue.
- **Regulation and ethics:** The development of new drugs through biotechnology also raises important ethical and regulatory issues. Regulatory agencies must assess not only the efficacy but also the safety of new treatments before they are approved for market.

3. **Genetic engineering in biotechnology**

Genetic engineering, an essential branch of biotechnology, involves the direct manipulation of an organism's genes. The discipline has evolved rapidly since its beginnings in the 1970s, when scientists began using restriction enzymes to cut DNA and insert genes of interest into plasmid vectors. Today, genetic engineering is applied in a variety of fields, including agriculture, medicine and industry.

Fundamental principles of genetic engineering: Genetic engineering is based on several key techniques:

- **Gene cloning**: This involves isolating a specific gene and multiplying it in a suitable host.
- **Transgenesis**: This method introduces a foreign gene into the genome of an organism, creating a transgenic organism.

- **Genome editing**: Technologies like CRISPR-Cas9 enable precise modifications to genetic material, opening up new avenues for research and practical applications.

Agricultural applications

One of the most visible applications of genetic engineering is the creation of crops resistant to disease or harsh environmental conditions. For example, Bt corn has been modified to produce an insecticidal protein that protects against certain pests. These innovations aim to increase crop yields while reducing dependence on chemical pesticides.

Medical applications

In the medical field, genetic engineering plays a crucial role in the development of gene therapies to treat hereditary diseases. Researchers use this technology to correct mutations responsible for diseases such as cystic fibrosis or certain forms of cancer. It is also used to produce therapeutic proteins such as recombinant insulin.

Ethical and regulatory challenges

Despite its potential benefits, genetic engineering also raises ethical and regulatory concerns. Questions concerning food safety, environmental impacts and social implications are at the heart of public debate. Regulatory bodies need to establish clear guidelines to ensure that these technologies are used responsibly.

4. Omics methods

Omics methods, which encompass approaches such as genomics, transcriptomics, proteomics and metabolomics, have become essential tools in modern biological sciences. These methods enable exhaustive analysis of biomolecules at different levels of biological organization, providing an integrated understanding of complex biological systems.

a. Genomics

Genomics is a scientific discipline that focuses on the study of the genome, i.e. the entire genetic material of an organism. It encompasses various aspects, from the sequence of genes to their expression and function within biological systems. In-depth studies in genomics involve a detailed understanding of sequencing techniques, bioinformatics analysis, as well as clinical and environmental applications.

1) **Sequencing Techniques**
   DNA sequencing is at the heart of modern genomics. Methods such as Sanger sequencing, which was the first technique developed to determine DNA sequence, have been largely replaced by high-throughput sequencing (NGS) technologies. The latter enable millions of DNA fragments to be analyzed rapidly and efficiently, making it possible to sequence the entire genome of complex organisms.
2) **Bioinformatics**
   Analysis of the data generated by sequencing techniques requires expertise in bioinformatics. This includes the development of algorithms to assemble sequences, identify genetic variations (such as SNPs or single nucleotide polymorphisms), and analyze gene expression through methods such as RNA-Seq. Bioinformatics plays a crucial role in managing and interpreting the vast quantities of data generated by genomics experiments.
3) **Clinical Applications**
   Studies in genomics have led to significant advances in the medical field, particularly in the diagnosis and treatment of genetic diseases. For example, personalized medicine uses genomic information to tailor treatments to individual patient characteristics. Genetic tests can also predict susceptibility to certain diseases or help select the most effective therapies.
4) **Environmental Genomics**
   Genomics is not limited to human organisms; it is also being applied to the study of ecosystems and biodiversity. Metagenomics makes it possible to analyze genetic material recovered directly from environmental samples, providing insight into microbial diversity in different habitats without the need to grow these organisms in the laboratory.
5) **Ethics and Society**
   With the rapid advancement of genomics technologies, there is also a growing need to examine the ethical and societal implications associated with this research. Questions concerning the confidentiality of genetic data, informed consent for DNA testing, and the potential misuse of genetic information are raising important debate among scientists, legislators and citizens alike.

b. <u>Transcriptomics</u>

Transcriptomics is a scientific discipline that studies all the RNAs transcribed in a cell or organism at a given time. This approach makes it possible to analyze gene expression levels, understand regulatory mechanisms and explore the diversity of mRNA isoforms. In-depth transcriptomics studies involve the use of various techniques and technologies, including high-throughput sequencing (NGS), microarrays, and bioinformatics analysis.

1) **Sequencing Techniques**
   High-throughput sequencing has revolutionized transcriptomics by enabling the simultaneous sequencing of millions of RNA fragments. This offers unprecedented resolution for quantifying gene expression and identifying novel transcripts. Platforms such as Illumina and PacBio are widely used to generate transcriptomic data.
2) **Microarrays**
   Microarrays are another method used to study gene expression. They consist of microarrays containing specific probes which hybridize with target RNAs. Although less sensitive than high-throughput sequencing, they are still useful for targeted studies on specific gene sets.
3) **Bioinformatics analysis**
   Bioinformatics analysis is crucial in transcriptomics to process and interpret the vast quantities of data generated by sequencing or microarrays. Tools such as DESeq2 or EdgeR are used to normalize data and identify differentially expressed genes.
4) **Practical Applications**
   The practical applications of transcriptomics are vast, ranging from basic research into cell biology to clinical applications such as disease diagnosis or the development of targeted therapies. For example, transcriptome analysis can help identify biomarkers for certain pathologies such as cancer.
5) **Future challenges and prospects**
   Despite its advances, transcriptomics faces several challenges, including data complexity, biological variability between samples, and the need for rigorous experimental validation. In the future, the integration of multi-omics data (genomics, proteomics) could offer a more complete view of cellular function.

c. <u>Proteomics</u>

Proteomics is a scientific discipline that focuses on the study of proteins, in particular their structure, function, interactions and post-translational modifications. It is essential for understanding biological mechanisms at the cellular and molecular level. In-depth proteomics studies involve several advanced analytical techniques, including mass spectrometry, gel electrophoresis and high-performance liquid chromatography (HPLC). These methods can be used to identify and quantify proteins in various biological samples.

1) **Basic proteomics techniques:** The fundamental techniques used in proteomics include :

- **Mass spectrometry (MS)**: This method analyzes the mass of peptides generated by the enzymatic digestion of proteins. Mass spectrometry can be used to identify the proteins present in a complex sample, providing information on their molecular weight and structure.
- **Gel electrophoresis**: This technique separates proteins according to their size and electrical charge. Two-dimensional (2D) electrophoresis is particularly useful for analyzing complex mixtures of proteins.
- **Chromatography**: High-performance liquid chromatography (HPLC) is often used to purify proteins prior to analysis by mass spectrometry or electrophoresis.

2) **Proteomics applications**

Proteomics has a wide range of applications in many fields:

- **Cell biology**: By studying a cell's protein profile, researchers can better understand its metabolic pathways and regulatory mechanisms.
- **Medicine**: Proteomics plays a crucial role in the development of biomarkers for the early diagnosis of diseases, including cancer. Studies have shown that certain post-translational modifications can be associated with specific disease states.
- **Pharmacology**: Understanding the protein profile can help identify new therapeutic targets and develop more effective drugs.

3) **Challenges in proteomics:** Despite its advances, proteomics faces several challenges:

- **Proteome complexity**: The sheer number of proteins expressed in an organism, along with their isoforms and post-translational modifications, makes analysis a complex task.
- **Accurate quantification**: Although methods such as mass spectrometry are powerful, obtaining accurate quantification of proteins remains a challenge due to natural biological variations.

4) **Future prospects**

The future of proteomics looks promising with the advent of new technologies such as artificial intelligence and machine learning, which could improve the analysis of the massive data generated by proteomic experiments. In addition, integration with other omics (genomics, transcriptomics) could provide a more comprehensive overview of biological functioning.

d. Metabolomics

Metabolomics is a scientific discipline that focuses on the study of metabolites, i.e. the small molecules produced during metabolic processes in living organisms. This branch of systems biology makes it possible to analyze the metabolic profiles of biological samples, such as blood, urine or tissue, in order to understand the biological mechanisms underlying various physiological and pathological conditions.

1) **Definition and Importance of Metabolomics**
   Metabolomics is often defined as the quantitative and qualitative analysis of metabolites in a given sample. These metabolites can include amino acids, fatty acids, sugars, nucleotides and other small molecules. The importance of metabolomics lies in its ability to provide an overview of the biological status of an organism at a given point in time. Indeed, unlike genomics or transcriptomics, which focus on DNA and RNA respectively, metabolomics offers direct insight into the end products of metabolism.
2) **Techniques used in metabolomics:** Metabolomics studies rely on several advanced analytical techniques:

- **Mass spectrometry (MS)**: This technique measures the mass of molecules and identifies the compounds present in a sample.
- **Gas chromatography (GC)**: Used to separate volatile compounds prior to analysis by mass spectrometry.
- **High-Performance Liquid Chromatography (HPLC)**: Enables the separation and analysis of non-volatile compounds.
- **Nuclear Magnetic Resonance (NMR)**: Provides structural information on the molecules present in a sample.
- These techniques are often combined to obtain a more complete and precise analysis of metabolic profiles.

3) **Practical applications of Metabolomics:** Metabolomics has found applications in various fields:

- **Medicine**: It is used to identify biomarkers associated with certain diseases, enabling early diagnosis or a better understanding of disease progression.
- **Nutrition**: Metabolomics studies can help us understand how different foods affect the human metabolic profile.
- **Pharmacology**: Research into pharmacological effects can benefit from analysis of changes in the metabolic profile following drug administration.

4) **Future challenges and prospects**
   Despite its advantages, metabolomics faces several challenges:

- **Data complexity**: The interpretation of data generated by analytical techniques can be complex due to the large number of variables involved.

- **Standardization**: There is still an urgent need for standardized protocols to ensure that results are comparable between different studies.
  In the future, with continued technological progress and the development of more sophisticated analytical algorithms, it is likely that metabolomics will play an even more crucial role in our understanding of human and animal biology.

e. Omics data integration

The integration of omics data is a rapidly expanding field that plays a crucial role in modern biology, personalized medicine and biomedical research. The term "omics" refers to a series of scientific disciplines that study the complete sets of molecules in an organism, including the genome (genomics), transcriptome (transcriptomics), proteome (proteomics) and metabolome (metabolomics). Integrating these different layers of information enables a more holistic understanding of biological systems.

1. Fundamental concepts: omics data integration is based on several key concepts:

- **Multidisciplinarity**: omics approaches require collaboration between various disciplines such as biology, bioinformatics, statistics and engineering.
- **Big Data**: Modern technologies generate huge quantities of data. Analyzing and interpreting this data requires advanced data management and analysis tools.
- **Systems modeling**: The integration of omics data enables the construction of systems models that can predict biological behavior based on the interaction between different molecules.

2. Integration methods: There are several methods for integrating omics data:

- **Network-based approaches**: These methods use graphs to represent interactions between different types of molecules. For example, protein-protein networks can be used to understand how proteins interact in a given biological context.
- **Multivariate statistical analysis**: techniques such as principal component analysis (PCA) or discriminant analysis are often used to reduce the dimensionality of data while preserving their informative structure.

- **Machine learning**: Machine learning algorithms are applied to identify complex patterns in integrated data sets.

3. Practical applications: The practical applications of omics data integration are vast:

- **Personalized medicine**: By integrating genetic, proteomic and metabolomic information, it is possible to develop treatments tailored to a patient's specific characteristics.
- **Biomarker discovery**: The identification of biomarkers associated with certain diseases can be facilitated by the integration of different omics layers.
- **Cancer research**: In the field of cancer, the integration of omics data helps to understand tumor complexity and develop targeted therapies.

4. Challenges: Despite its advantages, omics data integration presents several challenges:

- **Data heterogeneity**: Different data sources can vary considerably in terms of quality and format.
- **Biological interpretation**: Translating the results of integrated analysis into usable biological knowledge remains a complex task.
- **Ethical issues**: Collecting and using large quantities of biological data also raises ethical concerns about confidentiality and consent.

5. Clinical trials and regulations

Clinical trials are research studies conducted on human participants to evaluate the efficacy and safety of a new treatment or drug. They follow a rigorous process, often divided into several phases, each with specific objectives.

Clinical trial phases

- **Phase I**: This phase involves a small number of participants (usually between 20 and 100) and aims to assess the drug's safety, determine an appropriate dose and identify potential side effects. Researchers carefully monitor participants for any adverse reactions.

- **Phase II**: Once the drug has been deemed safe in Phase I, it moves on to Phase II, where it is administered to a larger group (around 100 to 300 people) to assess its efficacy against the targeted disease, while continuing to monitor its safety.

- **Phase III**: This phase involves thousands of participants (often several thousand) and compares the new treatment with the standard treatment or a placebo. The main aim is to confirm the drug's efficacy, analyze side effects and gather information that will enable researchers to understand how the drug works in a wider population.

- **Phase IV**: Following approval by the regulatory authorities, the drug can be marketed. Phase IV consists of post-marketing surveillance to detect any rare or long-term side effects not observed in previous phases.

Regulations

Regulation of clinical trials is essential to ensure that studies are conducted ethically and scientifically. Bodies such as the Food and Drug Administration (FDA) in the United States or the European Medicines Agency (EMA) in Europe set strict guidelines concerning :

- Test design
- Informed consent of participants
- Protecting the rights and well-being of subjects
- Transparent communication of results

Ethics committees also play a crucial role in reviewing and approving clinical trial protocols before they are implemented.

Ethical importance

Ethics in clinical trials is paramount to ensure that the rights and welfare of participants are protected. This includes respect for informed consent, where participants must be fully informed about potential risks and benefits before taking part in the study.

6. Ethical and social challenges in biotechnology

Biotechnology, which encompasses a wide range of techniques that use living organisms or their systems to develop or create products, raises numerous ethical and social challenges. These challenges are of crucial importance as they affect public health, the environment, the economy and human rights. In-depth studies in this field focus on several key aspects:

1. Ethics of genetic manipulation

One of the main ethical challenges in biotechnology is genetic manipulation, particularly in the context of genetic engineering and gene editing (such as CRISPR). Questions that arise include: Who has the right to modify genes? What are the potential risks for biodiversity? Could genetic modification lead to greater social inequalities if it is not accessible to all?

2. Social consequences of GMOs

Genetically modified organisms (GMOs) are generating intense debate about their food safety, their impact on traditional agriculture and their effects on rural communities. Concerns include the increased dependence of farmers on large biopharmaceutical companies and the economic implications for small-scale farmers.

3. Human rights and access to technology

Another major challenge is related to human rights, particularly with regard to equitable access to biotechnology technologies. This raises questions about social justice: how can we ensure that advances in biotechnology benefit everyone, including marginalized populations?

4. Regulation and governance

Biotechnology regulation is complex and varies considerably from country to country. Governance issues include: How do we establish ethical standards for biotechnology research? What role do ethics committees play in the decision-making process? Transparency in the development and application of technologies is essential to maintain public trust.

5. Environmental impact

The environmental implications of biotechnology are also an important subject of study. The use of modified organisms can have unforeseen effects on local ecosystems, including the possibility of undesirable effects on non-target species or the ecosystem as a whole.

Practical work: The Role of Modifier Genes in Sickle Cell Syndrome: A Therapeutic Perspective

Introduction

Sickle cell syndrome, also known as sickle cell anemia, is an inherited genetic disorder caused by a mutation in the beta-globin gene. This condition leads to the formation of sickle-shaped red blood cells, which can cause a variety of health problems, including pain, infection and organ complications. Modifier genes play a crucial role in the phenotypic variability observed in patients with this disease. This practical work aims to explore the impact of modifier genes on sickle cell syndrome and discuss the therapeutic prospects they offer.

1. Understanding Sickle Cell Syndrome

Sickle cell syndrome results primarily from a mutation in the HBB gene, which codes for the hemoglobin beta chain. However, other genes can influence the severity and clinical manifestations of the disease. These modifier genes can affect fetal hemoglobin (HbF) production, inflammation and other biological processes.

2. Identification of modifier genes

Studies have identified several modifier genes that influence the phenotype of sickle cell syndrome:

- **HBG1 and HBG2**: These genes code for fetal hemoglobin gamma chains, an increase in which can reduce symptoms.
- **BCL11A**: This transcription factor inhibits the expression of fetal hemoglobin genes; its regulation could be a therapeutic target.
- **KLF1**: Another transcription factor involved in globin regulation.

3. Mechanisms of action: modifier genes often act through complex mechanisms such as :

- **Increased HbF**: HbF has a protective effect against the harmful effects of hemoglobin S (HbS).
- **Inflammatory regulation**: Certain modulating genes can influence inflammatory pathways, thereby reducing painful attacks.

4. Therapeutic prospects: The identification and understanding of modifier genes opens up several therapeutic avenues:

- **Gene therapies**: Modify or replace the genes responsible to increase HbF expression.
- **Pharmacological inhibitors**: Develop drugs targeting BCL11A or KLF1 to stimulate HbF production.
- **Stem cell transplantation**: Using this approach to treat severe cases by replacing diseased blood cells with healthy ones.

Conclusion

Modifier genes represent an essential dimension in our understanding of the sickle cell syndrome, and offer significant potential for the development of new therapeutic strategies. By integrating this knowledge into clinical practice, it is possible to significantly improve the quality of life of affected patients.

Chapter 2: Immunotherapy

Introduction

Immunotherapy is a therapeutic approach that uses the body's immune system to fight disease, particularly cancer. Unlike traditional treatments such as chemotherapy and radiotherapy, which directly target tumor cells, immunotherapy aims to strengthen or restore the immune system's natural ability to recognize and destroy cancer cells.

A. Immune mechanisms

In-depth, hands-on studies of immune mechanisms encompass a wide range of research and applications aimed at understanding how the immune system functions, interacts with pathogens, and maintains homeostasis in the body. The immune system is a complex network of cells, tissues and organs that work together to defend the body against infection, disease and other threats.

1. Components of the Immune System

The immune system is divided into two main categories: innate and adaptive immunity. Innate immunity is the first line of defense against infection. It comprises physical barriers (such as the skin), phagocytic cells (such as macrophages), and plasma proteins (such as complement). Adaptive immunity, on the other hand, is specific to previously encountered pathogens, and involves the production of antibodies by B lymphocytes and the response of T lymphocytes.

2. Recognition mechanisms

Recognition mechanisms are crucial to the functioning of the immune system. Pattern recognition receptors (PRRs) on immune cells detect molecular motifs associated with pathogens (PAMPs) or danger signals (DAMPs). This recognition triggers a cascade of events leading to an appropriate immune response.

3. Immune response

The immune response can be divided into several stages: activation, proliferation, differentiation and memory. When a pathogen is recognized, antigen-presenting cells (APCs) activate naive T lymphocytes, which then multiply and differentiate into effector cells capable of eliminating the infection, or memory cells that provide long-term protection.

4. Practical applications

Knowledge of immune mechanisms has led to practical applications in diverse fields such as vaccination, cancer immunotherapy and the development of biological drugs. For example, vaccines exploit immunological memory to prepare the body to fight future infections without causing disease.

5. Current Research

Current research is also exploring how the human microbiome influences the immune system, as well as the implications of immune system dysfunction in various autoimmune and allergic diseases. Studies are being conducted to better understand how to modulate these responses to improve human health.

1. The physical barrier in innate immunity

Innate immunity is the body's first line of defense against pathogens. It consists of physical, chemical and biological barriers that prevent microbes from entering the body. Physical barriers play a crucial role in this early immune response.

Physical barriers: Physical barriers include the skin, mucous membranes and airway cilia. The skin is a robust barrier that prevents the penetration of pathogens thanks to its multilayered structure. Mucous membranes, found in the respiratory, digestive and urogenital systems, secrete mucus that traps foreign particles and contains antimicrobial enzymes.

- **Skin**: The horny layer of the epidermis is rich in keratin, making it difficult for microbes to penetrate this barrier. What's more, the skin has a resident microbial flora that can inhibit the growth of pathogens.

- **Mucous membranes**: Mucous membranes secrete mucus, which captures pathogens. In the respiratory system, for example, mucus is transported by cilia to the throat, where it can be expelled or swallowed.

- **Microbial flora**: The presence of commensal bacteria on the skin and in the intestinal tract also contributes to innate immunity by occupying ecological niches that might otherwise be colonized by pathogens.

Diseases Associated with Physical Barrier Failures: When these barriers are compromised, it can lead to a variety of infectious diseases. For example:

- **Skin infections**: A cut or burn can allow bacteria to enter the body.

- **Respiratory infections**: Impaired mucociliary function can lead to mucus build-up and promote infection by viruses or bacteria.
- **Gastrointestinal diseases**: altered intestinal flora (dysbiosis) can make the host more susceptible to infections such as those caused by Clostridium difficile.

Treatments : Treatment of diseases resulting from physical barrier failure often depends on the type of infection:

- **Antibiotics**: Used to treat bacterial infections when the skin or other barriers are compromised.
- **Antivirals**: Prescribed to treat certain viral infections when the respiratory tract is affected.
- **Probiotics**: Used to restore healthy intestinal flora after an imbalance caused by antibiotic treatment or illness.

In addition, there are also preventive approaches such as vaccines that boost the immune system against certain pathogens before they have a chance to bypass these physical barriers.

2. Immune cells

Immune cells play a crucial role in the body's defense against infection and disease. Studying them in depth involves understanding the different cell types and their functions, as well as the diseases that can result from immune dysfunction and the treatments available.

In-depth studies of immune cells

Immune cells fall into two main categories: innate and adaptive. The former include macrophages, neutrophils and dendritic cells, which react rapidly to pathogens. The latter include B and T lymphocytes, responsible for immune memory and antigen-specific response.

- **Innate cells**: These cells are the first line of defense. Macrophages phagocytose (ingest) pathogens, while neutrophils release enzymes to destroy these foreign agents. Dendritic cells play a key role in activating T lymphocytes by presenting antigens.

- **Adaptive cells**: B lymphocytes produce specific antibodies that neutralize pathogens, while cytotoxic T lymphocytes directly destroy infected or cancerous cells. Immune memory is essential for a rapid response to subsequent exposure to the same pathogen.

Diseases linked to the immune system: Diseases can occur when the immune system is either too active (autoimmune diseases) or not active enough (immunodeficiencies).

- **Auto-immune diseases**: In these conditions, the immune system mistakenly attacks its own tissues. Examples include systemic lupus erythematosus and multiple sclerosis.

- **Immunodeficiencies**: These can be congenital (such as Combined Immunodeficiency Syndrome) or acquired (such as HIV/AIDS), where the body cannot fight infections effectively.

Treatments : The treatment of immune-related diseases varies according to the nature of the disease:

- **Immunosuppressants**: used in autoimmune diseases to reduce the activity of the immune system.

- **Biological therapies**: These treatments specifically target certain immune system pathways to treat conditions such as rheumatoid arthritis or certain cancers.

- **Vaccines**: They stimulate the immune system to recognize and fight specific pathogens without causing disease.

- **Gene therapies**: Under study to treat certain forms of immunodeficiency by correcting or replacing defective genes.

- **Stem cell transplantation**: Used to treat certain forms of severe immunodeficiency by restoring a functional immune system.

3. Chemical mediators

Chemical mediators play a crucial role in innate immunity, the body's first line of defense against pathogens. These mediators, which include cytokines, chemokines, acute phase proteins and other signaling molecules, are essential for orchestrating the immune response and regulating inflammation. In this in-depth review, we will examine the different types of chemical mediators, their mechanism of action in innate immunity, their involvement in various diseases and associated treatments.

1. Types of Chemical Mediators: Chemical mediators can be classified into several categories:

- **Cytokines**: These are proteins produced by immune cells that modulate the immune response. Interleukins (IL), tumor necrosis factors (TNF) and interferons (IFN) are among the best known.

- **Chemokines**: These small proteins direct the movement of immune cells to the site of infection or inflammation.

- **Acute Phase Proteins**: Synthesized mainly by the liver in response to inflammation, they include C-reactive protein (CRP) and fibrinogen.

- **Lipid mediators**: eicosanoids such as prostaglandins and leukotrienes derived from polyunsaturated fatty acids also play a key role in inflammation.

2. Mechanisms of action: Chemical mediators act by binding to specific receptors on target cells, triggering a cascade of intracellular signals. For example:

- Cytokines such as TNF-α can induce apoptosis (programmed cell death) in certain infected cells.

- Chemokines attract neutrophils and other leukocytes to the site of infection, creating a chemical gradient.

- These interactions are essential for a rapid and effective response to infections.

3. Involvement in disease: Dysregulation of chemical mediators can lead to a variety of diseases:

- **Auto-immune diseases**: Excessive production of pro-inflammatory cytokines can contribute to conditions such as rheumatoid arthritis or systemic lupus erythematosus.

- **Allergies** : Mediators such as histamine play a central role in allergic reactions.

- **Infectious diseases**: an inappropriate inflammatory response can lead to tissue damage during viral or bacterial infections.

4. Associated treatments : Understanding the role of chemical mediators has led to the development of targeted treatments:

- **Cytokine inhibitors**: Drugs like adalimumab specifically target certain cytokines to treat autoimmune diseases.

- **Antihistamines**: Used to treat allergies by blocking the action of histamine.

- **Immunomodulatory therapies**: These treatments aim to restore a balance in the production of chemical mediators to alleviate excessive or insufficient inflammation.

4. Adaptive immunity

a) B lymphocytes

B lymphocytes play a central role in adaptive immunity, which is the specific immune response to pathogens. Unlike innate immunity, which is the first line of defense against infection, adaptive immunity is characterized by its ability to recognize specific antigens and develop an immunological memory. B lymphocytes are responsible for producing antibodies, which are proteins capable of neutralizing pathogens or marking them for destruction by other immune system cells.

1. B lymphocyte development and activation

B lymphocytes develop in the bone marrow and undergo several stages of maturation before being released into the bloodstream. When a B lymphocyte encounters a specific antigen, it can be activated with the help of T helper lymphocytes. This activation leads to the proliferation of B lymphocytes and their differentiation into plasma cells, which secrete antibodies. B lymphocytes can also form memory cells, enabling a more rapid response when re-exposed to the same antigen.

2. Role in diseases

B-cell dysfunction can lead to various autoimmune diseases, where the immune system attacks healthy body tissues. For example, in systemic lupus erythematosus (SLE), B lymphocytes produce autoantibodies that target the body's own cells and tissues. In addition, some forms of cancer, such as non-Hodgkin's lymphoma or chronic lymphocytic leukemia, involve abnormal proliferation of B lymphocytes.

3. Treatments targeting B lymphocytes

Treatment of diseases linked to B-cell dysfunction may include the use of biological agents such as monoclonal antibodies. These treatments specifically target malignant B cells, or regulate their activity in the case of autoimmune diseases. For example, rituximab is a monoclonal antibody used to treat certain types of blood cancer, as well as certain autoimmune diseases, by targeting CD20 on B cells.

4. Current search

Research continues to explore how to modulate the activity of B lymphocytes to improve treatments for various diseases. Studies focus on genetic manipulation to create B-cell lines capable of producing specific therapeutic antibodies, or on the development of vaccines that exploit the immunological memory induced by these cells.

b) T lymphocytes

T lymphocytes play a central role in adaptive immunity, which is the body's specific, long-term immune response against pathogens. These cells are derived from hematopoietic stem cells in the bone marrow and undergo maturation in the thymus, where they acquire specific receptors called T cell receptors (TCRs). T lymphocytes fall into two main categories: helper T lymphocytes (CD4+) and cytotoxic T lymphocytes (CD8+), each with distinct but complementary functions.

T cell function

- **Activation**: T-cell activation requires specific recognition of the antigen presented by antigen-presenting cells (APCs) via the major histocompatibility complex (MHC). CD4+ T cells recognize antigens presented by MHC class II, while CD8+ T cells recognize those presented by MHC class I.

- **Proliferation and differentiation**: Once activated, T lymphocytes proliferate and differentiate into effector subtypes. CD4+ T lymphocytes can transform into different types of helper cells (Th1, Th2, Th17, etc.), each playing a specific role in regulating the immune response. CD8+ T lymphocytes become cytotoxic cells capable of directly destroying infected or tumoral cells.

- **Immunological memory**: Once the pathogen has been eliminated, some T lymphocytes persist as memory cells. These cells enable a rapid, effective response when re-exposed to the same antigen.

Role in diseases: T-cell dysfunction can contribute to a variety of diseases:

1. **Autoimmune diseases**: In these conditions, such as systemic lupus erythematosus or multiple sclerosis, inappropriate activation or altered tolerance of T lymphocytes can lead to an attack on healthy tissue.

2. **Viral infections**: Chronic infections with certain viruses such as HIV can deplete or alter T-cell function, making the individual more vulnerable to opportunistic infections.

3. **Cancer**: Tumors can develop mechanisms to evade T-cell-mediated immune surveillance. However, immunotherapy targeting these cells has emerged as a promising treatment for various cancers.

Treatments: T-cell-based treatment includes several approaches:

- **Immunotherapy**: Treatments such as immune checkpoint inhibitors (like pembrolizumab) increase T-cell activity against tumors.

- **Cell-based therapies**: CAR-T therapy involves genetically modifying the patient's T lymphocytes so that they express a chimeric receptor capable of specifically recognizing and attacking cancer cells.

- **Therapeutic vaccines**: These vaccines aim to stimulate a specific immune response against certain infectious diseases or cancers by effectively activating T lymphocytes.

B. Therapeutic vaccines

Therapeutic vaccines against viral infections represent a promising approach in the field of immunotherapy. Unlike prophylactic vaccines, which aim to prevent infection before it occurs, therapeutic vaccines are designed to treat established infections by boosting the host's immune response.

Mechanisms of action of therapeutic vaccines: Therapeutic vaccines act primarily through the following mechanisms:

- **Stimulation of the immune response**: These vaccines are formulated to specifically activate T and B lymphocytes, which play a crucial role in recognizing and eliminating virus-infected cells. For example, some vaccines use viral peptides to induce a TCD8+ (cytotoxic T lymphocyte) response capable of destroying infected cells.

- **Production of neutralizing antibodies**: Vaccines can also induce the production of antibodies that bind to viruses and prevent their entry into host cells. This is particularly relevant in the case of viral infections such as HIV or hepatitis C.

- **Immune system education**: Therapeutic vaccines can educate the immune system to recognize specific antigens associated with viruses, which can help control or eliminate infection.

- **Use of viral or non-viral vectors**: Some vaccines use vectors (such as modified viruses) to carry viral antigens into the body to stimulate a robust immune response.

- **Adjuvants** : The addition of adjuvants can enhance the immune response by increasing antigen presentation and activating various types of immune cells.

List of Therapeutic Vaccines Against Viral Infections: Here are some examples of therapeutic vaccines currently under development or in use:

- **HIV vaccine (HIV-1)**: Uses peptides or viral vectors to induce a targeted immune response against HIV.

- **Hepatitis B vaccine (HBV)**: DNA- and recombinant protein-based approaches are used to stimulate an immune response in chronically infected patients.

- **Hepatitis C vaccine (HCV)**: Clinical trials are exploring various vaccine candidates aimed at generating an effective T cell response.

- **HPV (Human Papillomavirus) cancer vaccine**: Although primarily preventive, some treatments aim to treat early lesions caused by HPV by stimulating an immune response.

- **Cytomegalovirus (CMV) vaccine**: Studies are underway into a vaccine that could reduce CMV reactivation in immunocompromised individuals.

1. Tumor antigens

Therapeutic vaccines against tumor antigens represent a promising approach to the treatment of cancer. Unlike prophylactic vaccines, which aim to prevent disease by stimulating an immune response prior to exposure to a pathogen, therapeutic vaccines are designed to treat established diseases, particularly cancer. These vaccines exploit the immune system's ability to recognize and attack tumor cells by targeting specific tumor-associated antigens.

How therapeutic vaccines work

- **Tumor Antigen Identification**: Tumor antigens can be classified into two main categories: tumor-specific antigens (TSA), which are expressed only by cancer cells, and tumor-associated antigens (TAA), which may also be present in normal cells but are overexpressed in tumors. TSA and TAA serve as targets for the vaccine.

- **Immune system activation**: Therapeutic vaccines typically contain peptides or proteins derived from tumor antigens, often combined with an adjuvant to boost the immune response. When administered, these components stimulate an adaptive immune response, resulting in the production of cytotoxic T lymphocytes capable of recognizing and destroying cancer cells expressing these antigens.

- **Immunological memory**: A key aspect of vaccines is their ability to induce immunological memory. This means that the immune system can remember the tumor antigen and respond more quickly and effectively to future exposure.

List of Therapeutic Tumor Antigen Vaccines

1. **Sipuleucel-T (Provenge)**: Used to treat castration-resistant metastatic prostate cancer. This vaccine is made from the patient's own dendritic cells, which are activated with a prostate-specific antigen (PAP) before being reintroduced into the body.

2. **GVAX**: A vaccine based on cancer cells genetically modified to express specific tumor antigens while secreting stimulatory cytokines to attract and activate T lymphocytes.

3. **OncoVax**: For the treatment of melanoma, this vaccine uses a mixture of tumor antigens extracted from the patient's tumor to stimulate a specific immune response against it.

4. **NY-ESO-1 Vaccine**: Targeting the NY-ESO-1 antigen, this vaccine has shown efficacy in several types of cancer, including melanoma and non-small cell lung cancer.

5. **DCVAC**: A dendritic cell-based vaccine designed to treat colorectal cancer by presenting various tumor antigens to T lymphocytes to induce a targeted immune response against the tumor.

2. Viral infections

Therapeutic vaccines against viral infections represent a promising approach in the field of immunotherapy. Unlike prophylactic vaccines, which aim to prevent infection before it occurs, therapeutic vaccines are designed to treat established infections by boosting the host's immune response.

Mechanisms of action of therapeutic vaccines: Therapeutic vaccines act primarily through the following mechanisms:

- **Stimulation of the immune response**: These vaccines are formulated to specifically activate T and B lymphocytes, which play a crucial role in recognizing and eliminating virus-infected cells. For example, some vaccines use viral peptides to induce a TCD8+ (cytotoxic T lymphocyte) response capable of destroying infected cells.

- **Production of neutralizing antibodies**: Vaccines can also induce the production of antibodies that bind to viruses and prevent their entry into host cells. This is particularly relevant in the case of viral infections such as HIV or hepatitis C.

- **Immune system education**: Therapeutic vaccines can educate the immune system to recognize specific antigens associated with viruses, which can help control or eliminate infection.

- **Use of viral or non-viral vectors**: Some vaccines use vectors (such as modified viruses) to carry viral antigens into the body to stimulate a robust immune response.

- **Adjuvants** : The addition of adjuvants can enhance the immune response by increasing antigen presentation and activating various types of immune cells.

List of Therapeutic Vaccines Against Viral Infections: Here are some examples of therapeutic vaccines currently under development or in use:

1. **HIV vaccine (HIV-1)**: Uses peptides or viral vectors to induce a targeted immune response against HIV.

2. **Hepatitis B vaccine (HBV**): DNA- and recombinant protein-based approaches are used to stimulate an immune response in chronically infected patients.

3. **Hepatitis C vaccine (HCV**): Clinical trials are exploring various vaccine candidates aimed at generating an effective T cell response.

4. **HPV (Human Papillomavirus) cancer vaccine**: Although primarily preventive, some treatments aim to treat early lesions caused by HPV by stimulating an immune response.

5. **Cytomegalovirus (CMV) vaccine**: Studies are underway into a vaccine that could reduce CMV reactivation in immunocompromised individuals.

C. Cellular therapies such as CAR-T Cells

Cellular therapies represent a rapidly expanding field of research and application in the medical sector, aimed at treating various diseases through the use of living cells. These therapies may involve stem cells, modified immune cells, or other specific cell types that are manipulated to improve the patient's health.

1. Definition and Types of Cell Therapy: Cell therapies are defined as treatments that use cells to restore, replace or repair damaged tissues or organs. The main types include :

- **Stem cell therapy**: the use of stem cells to regenerate damaged tissue. Stem cells can be derived from a variety of sources, including embryos (embryonic stem cells) and adult tissues (adult stem cells).

- **Gene therapy**: Although distinct, it is often associated with cell therapy, as it involves the genetic modification of cells before they are reintroduced into the patient's body.

- **Immunotherapy**: Use of immune cells, such as modified T lymphocytes (like CAR-T), to target and destroy cancer cells.

2. Clinical applications: The clinical applications of cellular therapies are vast:

- **Oncology**: Treatments such as CAR-T therapy have shown remarkable efficacy in the treatment of certain types of leukemia and lymphoma.

- **Degenerative diseases**: Stem cell therapies show potential in the treatment of diseases such as Alzheimer's and multiple sclerosis.

- **Tissue regeneration**: In cases of serious injury or chronic disease, stem cell injections can promote healing and tissue regeneration.

3. Ethical and technical challenges: While promising, these therapies also raise a number of challenges:

- **Ethics**: The use of embryonic stem cells raises ethical questions about the moral status of embryos.

- **Safety and efficacy**: Cell manipulation can entail risks such as immune rejection or tumor formation.

4. Future prospects

The future of cell-based therapies looks bright with technological advances in cell biology and tissue engineering. Research continues to explore ways of optimizing these treatments to make them safer and more effective.

1. Cell biology and its mechanisms of action

Cell biology is a fundamental branch of biology that focuses on the study of cells, their structure, function, interactions and mechanisms of action. It plays a crucial role in our understanding of biological processes at all levels, from the functioning of single-cell organisms to the complex systems of multicellular organisms.

1. Cell structure

Cells are considered the basic units of life. They possess various structures called organelles, each with a specific function. For example, the nucleus contains DNA and regulates cellular activities, while mitochondria are responsible for energy production through cellular respiration. The plasma membrane also plays an essential role in controlling the passage of substances in and out of the cell.

2. Mechanisms of Action

The mechanisms of action within cells include various biochemical processes such as cell signalling, cell division (mitosis and meiosis), and protein synthesis. Cell signaling enables cells to communicate with each other and respond to environmental stimuli. This often involves membrane receptors that detect external signals and trigger a cascade of intracellular reactions.

3. Cell Cycle

The cell cycle is a complex process comprising several phases: G1 (growth), S (DNA synthesis), G2 (preparation for division) and M (mitosis). Each phase is regulated by specific proteins called cyclins and cyclin-dependent kinases (CDKs). Errors in this cycle can lead to diseases such as cancer.

4. Cell Biology Techniques

Cell biology studies use a variety of techniques to observe and manipulate cells. These include electron microscopy, which provides a detailed view of cell structures, and cell culture techniques, which enable researchers to study cell behavior in a controlled environment.

5. Practical applications

The knowledge acquired through cell biology has practical applications in various fields such as medicine, where it contributes to the development of gene and cell therapies to treat various diseases. It also plays a key role in biomedical research to understand the mechanisms underlying human disease.

2. Clinical applications of cellular therapies

Cellular therapies represent a rapidly expanding field of regenerative medicine and clinical treatment. They involve the use of living cells to treat or prevent disease, focusing on the repair or replacement of damaged tissue. In-depth, practical studies of the clinical applications of cell-based therapies encompass many aspects, including the types of cells used, mechanisms of action, clinical indications, and associated ethical and regulatory challenges.

Types of Cells Used : Cell therapies can involve a variety of cell sources, including:

- **Stem cells**: These cells have the ability to differentiate into various cell types. Embryonic stem cells and adult stem cells (such as those found in bone marrow) are commonly studied.
- **Immune cells**: T-cell therapies such as CAR-T (Chimeric Antigen Receptor T-cell therapy) are used to treat certain cancers.
- **Somatic cells**: Patient-specific cells can be harvested, modified and reintroduced to treat conditions such as diabetes or certain heart diseases.

Mechanisms of Action: The mechanisms by which these therapies exert their therapeutic effect include :

- **Tissue repair**: Injected cells can migrate to the site of injury and promote tissue regeneration.
- **Immune modulation**: Some therapies target the immune system to reduce inflammation or improve the immune response against tumors.
- **Secretion of trophic factors**: Cells can secrete molecules that promote cell survival and proliferation.

Clinical indications: The clinical applications of cellular therapies are varied:

- **Oncology**: Innovative immunotherapy treatments for different types of cancer.
- **Degenerative diseases**: Use in conditions such as Alzheimer's or Parkinson's disease.

- **Cardiovascular pathologies**: repairing the heart muscle after a heart attack.

Ethical and regulatory challenges: The use of cell therapies also raises a number of ethical issues:

- **Informed consent**: The need for appropriate informed consent when using embryonic stem cells.
- **Regulation**: The need for a solid regulatory framework to guarantee the safety and efficacy of treatments.

3. Ethical and regulatory challenges in cell therapy

Cell-based therapies, which encompass innovative approaches such as stem cells, tissue engineering and immune cell-based treatments, represent a rapidly expanding field in regenerative medicine and disease treatment. However, these technological advances raise significant ethical and regulatory challenges that require careful attention.

Ethical Challenges

- **Informed Consent**: One of the key ethical challenges lies in the informed consent of patients. Cell therapies often involve the use of donor cells or embryonic tissue, raising questions about where these cells come from and whether patients understand the risks associated with these treatments.

- **Equity of Access**: Cell therapies can be expensive and are not always accessible to all patients. This poses an ethical dilemma concerning equity of access to advanced healthcare, where certain groups may be disadvantaged due to socio-economic factors.

- **Genetic manipulation**: With the advent of technologies such as CRISPR, genetic manipulation in the context of cell therapy raises ethical concerns about hereditary modifications and the implications for future generations.

- **Embryo use**: Research using embryonic stem cells gives rise to intense ethical debate concerning the moral status of the human embryo and the moral implications of destroying it to obtain these cells.

- **Clinical overpromise**: There is also a risk that some cell therapies are marketed with exaggerated promises of efficacy, which can mislead patients and compromise their well-being.

Regulatory challenges

- **Inadequate regulatory framework**: The rapid development of cell-based therapies has often outstripped the ability of regulatory bodies to establish an appropriate framework for their evaluation and approval. This can lead to variability in the quality and safety of treatments available on the market.

- **Manufacturing standards**: The manufacture of biological products such as cell therapies must comply with strict standards to guarantee their safety and efficacy. However, there are still gaps in the uniform implementation of these standards across different countries.

- **Post-marketing follow-up**: Once a cell therapy has been approved, it is crucial to ensure adequate follow-up to monitor its long-term effects on patients. This requires a robust infrastructure that is not always in place.

- **Intellectual property**: Intellectual property issues surrounding scientific discoveries in the field of cell therapy can hamper innovation, while raising ethical concerns about the right of access to treatments.

- **International collaboration**: Given that cell therapy research is conducted worldwide, it is essential to establish international collaboration to harmonize regulations to ensure adequate protection for clinical trial participants while fostering innovation.

4. Future prospects for cellular therapies

Cellular therapies represent a rapidly expanding field of research, offering promising prospects for the treatment of a variety of diseases, including degenerative diseases, cancers and immune disorders. These therapeutic approaches rely on the use of living cells to repair or replace damaged tissue, modulate the immune response or deliver drugs directly to target cells.

1. History and development of cell therapy

The history of cell therapy goes back several decades, with significant advances in our understanding of the role of stem cells and their therapeutic potential. The first clinical applications were observed in the context of bone marrow transplants to treat certain forms of leukemia. Since then, research has evolved towards the use of induced pluripotent stem (iPS) cells and other specialized cell types.

2. Types of cell therapy: Cell therapies can be classified into several categories:

- **Stem cell therapy**: Using embryonic or adult stem cells to regenerate tissue.
- **Cellular immunotherapy**: Use of modified T lymphocytes (such as CAR-T) to specifically target cancer cells.
- **Gene therapy**: Integrating genes into cells to correct genetic abnormalities.

3. Technological advances

Technological advances are playing a crucial role in the evolution of cellular therapies. Techniques such as CRISPR-Cas9 gene editing enable precise manipulation of the genome, paving the way for more targeted and effective treatments. In addition, bioengineering enables the development of three-dimensional matrices that support cell growth in vitro.

4. Ethical and regulatory challenges

Despite their promise, cell therapies also raise important ethical and regulatory challenges. Questions concerning the origin of stem cells, informed consent and long-term safety remain at the heart of scientific and public debate. Regulatory bodies need to establish clear guidelines to ensure that these treatments are safe and effective before they are put on the market.

5. Future prospects

The future of cellular therapies looks promising, thanks to ongoing research and technological innovation. Ongoing clinical studies are exploring the application of these treatments in various medical fields, including neurodegenerative diseases such as Alzheimer's or Parkinson's, as well as in the field of cellular aging. Personalizing treatments based on an individual's genetic profile could also transform the way we approach medical care.

Practical work: Identification of brain mechanisms linked to expertise and educational spin-offs

Introduction

Expertise in a particular field is often the result of years of deliberate practice, learning and experience. The brain mechanisms underlying this expertise are complex, involving several brain regions and specific cognitive processes. This practical work aims to explore these mechanisms and examine their implications for education.

Practical work objectives

- **Understanding the Neurological Basis of Expertise**: Students will research the different brain regions involved in the development of expertise, including the prefrontal cortex, motor cortex, and subcortical structures such as the striatum.

- **Analyzing Cognitive Processes Associated with Expertise**: It will be essential to explore how memory, attention and perception evolve with expertise. Students will need to identify how these processes are modulated by practice.

- **Examining the Educational Implications**: Students will be asked to consider the implications of these discoveries for teaching methods. How can teaching be adapted to take advantage of brain mechanisms linked to expertise?

Methodology

- **Bibliographic Research**: Students will use encyclopedias, academic books and scientific journal articles to gather information on the brain mechanisms associated with expertise.

- **Case study**: Each student chooses a field of expertise (music, sports, mathematics, etc.) and analyzes how neuroscientific research relates to this field.

- **Report writing**: At the end of the practical work, each student will be asked to write a report detailing his or her findings on brain mechanisms related to his or her chosen field, as well as his or her thoughts on the educational spin-offs.

- **Oral presentation**: Finally, each student will present his or her results to the class to encourage collective discussion on the subject.

Conclusion

This practical work will enable students not only to understand the neurological basis of expertise, but also to consider how this knowledge can be applied in an educational context to improve learning and performance.

Chapter 3: Gene therapy

Introduction

Gene therapy is an innovative and promising approach to medicine, aimed at treating or preventing disease by modifying an individual's genes. The technique is based on the idea that many diseases, particularly hereditary genetic diseases, are caused by abnormalities in a person's genetic material. By introducing, eliminating or modifying genes within a patient's cells, it is possible to correct these anomalies and thus improve the patient's health.

History and development

Gene therapy emerged in the 1970s with the first research into recombinant DNA. Scientists began to explore how healthy genes could be inserted into diseased cells to restore their normal function. The first gene therapy clinical trial took place in 1990, when researchers treated a young girl with a rare genetic disease called severe combined immunodeficiency (SCID). Although this trial was a limited success, it paved the way for many other studies and clinical trials.

Mechanisms of gene therapy: There are several approaches to gene therapy:

- **Gene insertion**: This involves introducing a functional gene into the patient's cells to replace a defective one.
- **Gene inhibition**: In some cases, it may be necessary to block the expression of a gene that contributes to a disease.
- **Genome editing**: Techniques such as CRISPR-Cas9 enable scientists to directly modify genetic material by targeting and modifying specific sequences.

Clinical applications: Gene therapy has shown significant potential in the treatment of a variety of conditions, including :

- Hereditary diseases such as cystic fibrosis and hemophilia.
- Cancers, where it can be used to boost the patient's immune system so that it can better fight cancer cells.
- Viral infections such as HIV.

Challenges and ethical considerations

Despite its promise, gene therapy also raises ethical and technical concerns. Potential risks include adverse immune reactions or off-target effects during genome editing. In addition, the ethical issues surrounding genetic modification in human embryos continue to be debated within the scientific community and the general public.

1. Viral and non-viral vectors

Viral and non-viral vectors are essential tools in biotechnology and medicine, particularly for the delivery of genes into target cells. Their in-depth study involves an understanding of the mechanisms underlying their function, as well as practical applications in fields such as gene therapy, vaccines and tissue engineering.

A. Viral vectors

Viral vectors are derived from viruses that have been modified to carry genetic material without causing disease. Common types of viral vector include :

1. DNA vectors :

DNA vectors, as biotechnology tools, play a crucial role in biomedical research and the development of gene therapies. These vectors are often used to introduce specific genes into cells in order to correct genetic abnormalities or induce an immune response against certain diseases. DNA vectors fall into several categories, including plasmids, modified viruses (such as lentiviruses and adenoviruses) and other delivery systems.

Diseases caused by DNA vectors: Although DNA vectors are mainly used to treat diseases, their use can also lead to complications. For example:

- **Immune reactions**: The introduction of a foreign vector may trigger an undesirable immune response in some patients, resulting in inflammation or an allergic reaction.

- **Mutagenic insertion**: The integration of foreign genetic material into the host genome can cause mutations that could lead to cancer or other genetic disorders.

- **Viral transmission**: Where a viral vector is used, there is a risk that the vector may replicate itself or transmit pathogens.

- **Inherited diseases**: Some approaches using DNA vectors have been associated with unforeseen side effects in patients with inherited diseases such as cystic fibrosis or certain forms of muscular dystrophy.

Treatments associated with DNA vectors: Treatments based on DNA vectors include:

1) **Gene therapy**: Gene therapy is an innovative approach to treating or preventing disease by introducing, modifying or deleting genes within a patient's cells. This technique relies on the use of DNA vectors, which are biological vehicles designed to transport genetic material into target cells. Vectors can be derived from viruses, but they can also be synthetic. The main aim of gene therapy is to correct genetic abnormalities responsible for hereditary diseases, to improve the immune response against cancers or to induce therapeutic effects in various pathologies.

   In-depth, hands-on studies

   - **Inherited diseases**: Gene therapy has shown significant potential in the treatment of genetic diseases such as cystic fibrosis, hemophilia and certain forms of muscular dystrophy. For example, in the case of hemophilia A, a viral vector can be used to introduce a gene coding for the missing factor VIII, enabling endogenous production of the factor and reducing bleeding episodes.
   - **Cancer**: In oncology, gene therapy is used to modify immune cells so that they recognize and attack tumor cells more effectively. DNA vectors can be used to introduce genes coding for immunostimulatory proteins, or to deactivate inhibitory genes in T lymphocytes.
   - **Neurodegenerative diseases**: Research is underway into the use of gene therapy to treat diseases such as Parkinson's and Alzheimer's. Here, DNA vectors can be used to deliver genes that promote neuronal survival or produce neurotrophic factors. Here, DNA vectors can be used to deliver genes that promote neuronal survival or produce neurotrophic factors.
   - **Cardiovascular disease**: Gene therapy can also play a role in the treatment of cardiovascular disease, by introducing genes that promote tissue regeneration or improve cardiac function after a heart attack.
   - **Viral infections**: Another promising area is the use of gene therapy to treat chronic viral infections such as HIV. Strategies

include the introduction of genes that code for antiviral proteins or modify cellular receptors to prevent viral entry.

DNA vectors: DNA vectors play a crucial role in these therapeutic applications:

- **Viral vectors**: These vectors are often derived from attenuated viruses (such as lentiviruses) capable of efficiently infecting human cells, but modified so as not to cause disease.
- **Non-viral vectors**: These include liposomes and other nanoparticle-based systems that enable safer delivery of genetic material without the use of infectious agents.

2) **DNA-based vaccines**:

Genetic vaccines, particularly those using DNA vectors, represent a significant advance in the field of vaccination and immunology. These vaccines work by introducing a DNA fragment that codes for an antigen specific to a pathogen, enabling the immune system to recognize and combat that pathogen upon future exposure. The use of DNA vectors offers several advantages, including stability, the ability to induce a robust immune response, and the possibility of being administered intramuscularly or intradermally.

Mechanism of action of DNA vaccines

DNA vaccines are designed to deliver plasmids containing the gene coding for the target antigen. Once injected into muscle or dendritic cells, the plasmid is transcribed and translated into an antigenic protein. This protein is then presented to the T and B cells of the immune system, triggering an adaptive immune response. This process can also include the activation of cytotoxic T lymphocytes, which are essential for eliminating infected cells.

Advantages of DNA vaccines

- **Stability**: DNA vectors are generally more stable than their RNA or protein counterparts, making them easier to store and transport.
- **Safety**: Since they do not contain live viruses, the risks associated with vaccine infection are considerably reduced.
- **Induction of a lasting immune response**: DNA vaccines can induce both humoral (antibodies) and cellular (T lymphocytes) responses, offering complete protection against infection.

Clinical applications

Genetic vaccines using DNA vectors have been explored in a variety of clinical contexts. For example, they have been used in the development of vaccines against diseases such as hepatitis B, HIV and, more recently, COVID-19. Clinical trials have shown that these vaccines can be effective while presenting a favorable safety profile.

Challenges and prospects

Despite their promising advantages, DNA vaccines face several technical challenges. The efficiency of plasmid delivery to target cells is crucial; various methods such as electroporation or the use of nanoparticles are currently being investigated to improve this step. In addition, there are still concerns about the potentially weak immune response in certain populations.

3) **Cancer treatments** :

Oncology, the branch of medicine that focuses on the diagnosis and treatment of cancer, has seen significant advances thanks to the use of DNA vectors. These vectors are essential tools in the research and development of gene therapies, enabling specific genes to be introduced into cancer cells to modify their behavior or destroy them. In-depth and practical studies in oncology using DNA vectors encompass several aspects, including vector design, mechanisms of action, clinical applications and associated challenges.

a. **DNA vector design**

DNA vectors can be derived from a variety of biological systems, including viruses (such as lentiviruses or adenoviruses) or bacterial plasmids. The design of these vectors requires a thorough understanding of the regulatory elements that control gene expression. Researchers need to ensure that the vector is able to enter target cells efficiently, while minimizing immunogenicity.

b. **Mechanisms of Action**

Once introduced into cancer cells, DNA vectors can perform several functions. For example, they can deliver pro-apoptotic genes that promote programmed cell death, or inhibit the expression of oncogenic genes responsible for tumor proliferation. In addition, some vectors are designed to produce therapeutic proteins that specifically target tumor cells.

c. **Clinical Applications**

Gene therapies based on DNA vectors have been tested in various clinical trials to treat different types of cancer. Trials have shown that these approaches can improve treatment response and prolong survival in patients with advanced cancers. For example, the use of viral vectors to deliver genes encoding immunostimulatory cytokines has shown promising potential in boosting the immune response against tumors.

d. Associated challenges

Despite their potential advantages, the use of DNA vectors in oncology presents several challenges. One of the main issues is the risk of random integration of genetic material into the host genome, which can lead to unwanted mutations or even promote carcinogenesis. There are also concerns about the long-term safety and efficacy of these treatments.

e. Future prospects

Ongoing research into the improvement of DNA vectors and their application in oncology is essential to develop safer and more effective cancer treatments. New technologies such as CRISPR-Cas9 also offer enormous potential for precisely targeting the genes involved in cancer, while reducing side effects.

4) **Epigenetic modifications**: Some researchers are exploring the use of vectors to modify gene expression without altering the DNA sequence itself, offering a new way of treating various diseases without the risk of mutagenic insertion.

5) **Tissue regeneration**: Vectors can also be used to introduce genes promoting cell regeneration as part of treatments for severe or degenerative injuries.

2. **RNA vectors** :

RNA vectors are essential tools in molecular biology and genetics. They play a crucial role in gene expression, gene therapy and gene functional studies. RNA vectors can be classified into several types, including messenger RNA (mRNA) vectors, interfering RNA (iRNA) vectors and RNA virus vectors.

a. Messenger RNA (mRNA) vectors

mRNA vectors are used to introduce DNA sequences coding for specific proteins into cells. These vectors are often derived from plasmids or viruses, and contain regulatory elements that enable efficient expression of the target gene. The use of these vectors is particularly important in the development of vaccines, such as those based on mRNA against COVID-19.

b. RNA interference vectors (RNAi)

RNAi vectors are designed to induce the targeted degradation of specific mRNAs by a mechanism known as RNA interference. This process is essential for studying gene function by enabling researchers to reduce the expression of a particular gene in a model organism. Applications include cancer research, where inhibition of oncogenic genes can provide insights into their role in tumor progression.

c. Viral vectors

Viral vectors, such as lentiviruses and adeno-associated viruses, are used to deliver DNA or RNA sequences into host cells. These systems are often used in gene therapy to correct genetic mutations responsible for hereditary diseases. Lentiviruses, for example, have the ability to transduce non-dividing cells, which extends their potential use.

d. Practical applications

The practical applications of RNA vectors extend beyond basic research. In the medical field, they are being used to develop innovative treatments for a variety of diseases, including infectious diseases and cancers. Moreover, with the advent of technologies such as CRISPR-Cas9, the combined use of RNA vectors with these tools enables precise and efficient genetic manipulation.

e. Ethical considerations

The growing use of RNA vectors also raises ethical questions concerning their application in human and animal medicine. The possibility of genetically modifying living organisms calls for strict regulations to ensure the safety and efficacy of proposed treatments.

Electroporation of non-viral vectors

Electroporation is a technique that uses electric fields to increase the permeability of cell membranes, enabling the introduction of molecules, such as nucleic acids, into cells. This method is particularly relevant in the context of non-viral vectors, which are often used for gene delivery due to their safety and relative efficacy compared to viral vectors.

- **Principles of electroporation:** Electroporation is based on the principle that the application of an electric field to a cell can induce the formation of transient pores in the plasma membrane. These pores allow macromolecules such as DNA or RNA to enter the cell without damaging its overall structure. The size and duration of the pores depend on several factors, including the intensity of the electric field, the duration of the pulse and the physical properties of the cell membrane.
- **Non-viral vector applications:** Non-viral vectors include liposomes, nanoparticles and other polymer-based systems. Electroporation is often used to facilitate their entry into cells. For example, liposomes can

encapsulate nucleic acids and be introduced into cells by electroporation, greatly enhancing transfection efficiency.

- **Advantages and disadvantages:**The main advantages of using electroporation with non-viral vectors include:
    - **Safety**: Unlike viral vectors, there is no risk of infection.
    - **Flexibility**: Researchers can easily modify formulations to optimize delivery.
    - **Effectiveness**: In some cases, electroporation can outperform traditional methods such as lipofection.

  However, there are also disadvantages:
    - **Cellular toxicity**: Electric fields that are too strong or too long can damage cells.
    - **Variability**: Efficacy may vary according to cell type and experimental conditions.
- **Future prospects:** Research continues to explore how to improve this technique to maximize its efficacy while minimizing its side effects. Recent studies are focusing on the development of standardized protocols for different cell types in order to standardize the results obtained by electroporation.

3. Retroviral vectors

Retroviral vectors are essential tools in molecular biology and gene therapy. They are derived from retroviruses, a class of virus that uses RNA as genetic material and can integrate this material into the genome of host cells. Studies on retroviral vectors focus mainly on their use to introduce therapeutic genes into target cells, with significant implications for the treatment of genetic diseases, cancers and viral infections.

a. Mechanism of action of retroviral vectors

Retroviral vectors work in a multi-step process. First, the virus must bind to the surface of the host cell via specific receptors. Once bound, the virus enters the cell and releases its viral RNA. This RNA is then converted into DNA by the enzyme reverse transcriptase, a key feature of retroviruses. The viral DNA is then integrated into the host cell genome by the integrase enzyme.

b. Types of retroviral vectors

There are several types of retroviral vector, including HIV (Human Immunodeficiency Virus)-based vectors, MLV (Murine Leukemia Virus)-

based vectors and lentiviral vectors. Each has its own advantages and disadvantages, depending on the desired application:

- **HIV-based vectors**: These vectors are capable of infecting non-dividing cells, which broadens their potential use.
- **MLV vectors**: Although less effective at infecting non-dividing cells, they are often used for their simplicity and safety.

c. Clinical applications

Clinical applications of retroviral vectors include gene therapy to correct genetic mutations responsible for hereditary diseases such as cystic fibrosis or certain forms of anemia. They are also being explored for cancer treatment, through the introduction of pro-apoptotic or immunomodulatory genes.

d. Challenges and ethical considerations

Despite their potential advantages, the use of retroviral vectors raises a number of technical and ethical challenges. These include the risks of random integration into the host genome, which can lead to oncogenic mutations or other undesirable effects. In addition, there is an ethical debate concerning genetic modification in humans.

e. Future prospects

Ongoing research into retroviral vectors aims to improve their efficacy and safety, while minimizing the risks associated with their clinical use. Innovative approaches such as the use of CRISPR/Cas9 combined with retroviral vectors could revolutionize gene therapy by enabling precise genome editing.

B. Non-Viral Vectors

Non-viral vectors offer an alternative to viral vectors and include several different methods:

1. **Liposomes**: Liposomes are spherical vesicular structures composed of one or more layers of phospholipids. They are used as non-viral vectors for the delivery of drugs, DNA and other biomolecules. Their design and use in biopharmaceuticals have attracted considerable interest due to their ability to encapsulate hydrophilic and hydrophobic substances, improve drug bioavailability, and specifically target tissues or cells.

a) Liposome structure and composition

Liposomes are mainly made up of phospholipids, which form a lipid bilayer similar to that of cell membranes. This structure enables liposomes to encapsulate active molecules in their aqueous core or in the lipid bilayer itself. Liposomes can be classified according to size (small unilamellar liposomes, large multilamellar liposomes) and lipid composition (neutral, cationic or anionic liposomes).

b) **Delivery mechanisms**

Liposomes act as non-viral vectors, facilitating targeted drug delivery. They can fuse with cell membranes, enabling the release of encapsulated contents directly into the cell cytoplasm. In addition, liposomes can be modified by adding specific ligands to their surface to enhance cellular targeting.

c) **Benefits of Liposomes**

- **Improved bioavailability**: liposomes increase the solubility and stability of hydrophobic drugs.
- **Reduced toxicity**: By encapsulating drugs, liposomes reduce systemic exposure to toxic agents.
- **Specific targeting**: Thanks to surface modifications, liposomes can specifically target certain cells or tissues.

d) **Clinical Applications**

- Liposomes are used in various clinical applications such as :
- Targeted chemotherapy to treat various types of cancer.
- Vaccination, where they are used as adjuvants to boost the immune response.
- Gene delivery, where they transport plasmid DNA to target cells.

e) **Future challenges and prospects**

Despite their advantages, the clinical use of liposomes presents certain challenges such as physical and chemical stability, control of drug release rate, and production cost. Ongoing research is aimed at overcoming these obstacles by developing more effective formulations and exploring new delivery methods.

2. **Nanoparticles**: Nanoparticles are nano-sized structures that have attracted considerable interest in biotechnology and medicine, particularly for their use as non-viral vectors in gene therapy and drug delivery. Unlike viral vectors, which can present risks of immunogenicity and toxicity, non-viral vectors offer a safer alternative for the transport of nucleic acids and other biomolecules.

   a. **Characteristics of nanoparticles**

Nanoparticles can be classified according to their composition (lipidic, polymeric, inorganic) and manufacturing method (top-down or bottom-up). Their small size gives them unique properties, such as a high specific surface area, which enhances adsorption of biological molecules. What's more, they can be chemically modified to enhance their cellular targeting and bioavailability.

b. Mechanisms of action

Non-viral vectors using nanoparticles generally work by endocytosis, where the cell engulfs the particles containing the genetic or therapeutic material. Entry mechanisms can vary according to the nature of the nanoparticles; for example, liposomes often promote membrane fusion, while polymeric nanoparticles can be internalized via specific receptors.

c. Clinical applications

Clinical applications of nanoparticles as non-viral vectors include gene therapy to treat various genetic diseases, as well as targeted delivery of anti-cancer drugs. Studies show that these systems can improve treatment efficacy while reducing the side effects associated with traditional chemotherapy.

d. Challenges and prospects

Despite their potential advantages, several challenges remain in the clinical use of nanoparticles as non-viral vectors. These include the need to optimize the formulation to ensure controlled release of the target drug or gene. In addition, it is crucial to overcome biological barriers such as the immune system and enzymatic degradation.

e. Future research

Ongoing research into nanoparticles focuses on improving their efficacy and safety through new design and engineering strategies. The integration of advanced technologies such as CRISPR genome editing with nanoparticle-based systems could open up new avenues for personalized disease treatment.

3. **Electroporation**: Electroporation is a technique that uses electric fields to increase the permeability of cell membranes, enabling the introduction of molecules, such as nucleic acids, into cells. This method is particularly relevant in the context of non-viral vectors, which are often used for gene delivery due to their safety and relative efficacy compared to viral vectors.

   Principles of electroporation: Electroporation is based on the principle that the application of an electric field to a cell can induce the formation of transient pores in the plasma membrane. These pores allow macromolecules such as DNA or RNA to enter the cell without damaging its overall structure. The size and duration of the pores depend on several factors, including the intensity of the electric field, the duration of the pulse and the physical properties of the cell membrane.

Non-viral vector applications: Non-viral vectors include liposomes, nanoparticles and other polymer-based systems. Electroporation is often used to facilitate their entry into cells. For example, liposomes can encapsulate nucleic acids and be introduced into cells by electroporation, greatly enhancing transfection efficiency.

Advantages and disadvantages : The main advantages of using electroporation with non-viral vectors include:

- **Safety**: Unlike viral vectors, there is no risk of infection.
- **Flexibility**: Researchers can easily modify formulations to optimize delivery.
- **Effectiveness**: In some cases, electroporation can outperform traditional methods such as lipofection.

However, there are also disadvantages:

- **Cellular toxicity**: Electric fields that are too strong or too long can damage cells.
- **Variability**: Efficacy may vary according to cell type and experimental conditions.

Future prospects

Research continues to explore how to improve this technique to maximize its efficacy while minimizing its side effects. Recent studies are focusing on the development of standardized protocols for different cell types in order to standardize the results obtained by electroporation.

4. **Micro-injection**: A direct method in which genetic material is injected directly into the cell nucleus using a fine micropipette.

2. Gene-editing techniques (CRISPR-Cas 9)

Gene editing is a revolutionary technique that enables the genome of an organism to be modified precisely and efficiently. Among the various gene-editing methods, the CRISPR-Cas9 system has emerged as one of the most promising due to its simplicity, flexibility and efficiency. This system is based on a natural immune mechanism observed in certain bacteria, which use CRISPR (Clustered Regularly Interspaced Short Palindromic Repeats) and Cas9 (CRISPR-associated protein 9) to defend themselves against viruses.

CRISPR-Cas9 mechanism

The CRISPR-Cas9 system is a revolutionary gene-editing technology that emerged from studies of bacterial immune systems. The term "CRISPR" stands for "Clustered Regularly Interspaced Short Palindromic Repeats", while "Cas" refers to the proteins associated with CRISPR. This system was discovered as a means by which bacteria protect themselves against viruses by integrating viral DNA sequences into their own genome, thus enabling an adaptive immune response.

Origins of CRISPR-Cas9: Research into the CRISPR system began in the 1980s, but it wasn't until the early 2000s that its role in bacterial defense was fully understood. Scientists discovered that bacteria could store viral DNA fragments in their CRISPR sequences, enabling them to recognize and target these viruses in subsequent infections. This discovery was key to understanding how the system functions as a gene-editing tool. **CRISPR-Cas9 mechanism:** The CRISPR-Cas9 mechanism is based on two main components: the guide RNA (gRNA) and the Cas9 protein. The guide RNA is designed to match a specific target DNA sequence in the genome of the organism to be modified. When the guide RNA associates with the Cas9 protein, it forms a complex that can bind to the target DNA. Once bound, Cas9 creates a double-strand break in the target DNA. This cut then triggers the cell's DNA repair mechanisms, which can be exploited to introduce specific modifications into the genome. Researchers can either insert a new gene or deactivate an existing one by exploiting these repair pathways.

CRISPR-Cas9 applications: The CRISPR-Cas9 system, a revolutionary gene-editing technology, has attracted considerable interest in the fields of biomedical research and medicine. Its development is based on fundamental discoveries in molecular biology, notably the immune mechanism of bacteria, which use CRISPR to defend themselves against viruses. This technology makes it possible to modify specific DNA sequences with remarkable precision, opening the way to a wide range of applications.

a. Operating mechanism

The CRISPR-Cas9 system works through two main components: the Cas9 enzyme and a guide RNA (gRNA). The guide RNA is designed to match a target DNA sequence in the genome. When the guide RNA binds to this sequence, the Cas9 enzyme is activated, creating a double-strand break in the DNA. This process then triggers the cell's natural DNA repair mechanisms, which can be exploited to introduce genetic modifications.

b. Research applications

In the field of research, CRISPR-Cas9 has been used to create genetically modified animal models to study human diseases. For example, it has enabled researchers to explore the mechanisms underlying cancer, neurodegenerative diseases such as Alzheimer's, and genetic disorders such as cystic fibrosis. By facilitating the study of the specific genes involved in these conditions, CRISPR-Cas9 has considerably accelerated our understanding of disease.

c. Medical applications

The clinical applications of CRISPR-Cas9 are also promising. Clinical trials are underway to evaluate its efficacy in the treatment of hereditary diseases such as sickle cell anemia and certain forms of hereditary blindness. In addition, this technology could potentially be used to treat certain viral infections by directly targeting the virus' genetic material.

d. Ethical and regulatory challenges

Despite its undeniable advantages, the use of CRISPR-Cas9 also raises significant ethical concerns. Questions concerning germline modifications (changes in DNA that can be passed on to future generations) are generating intense debate among scientists, ethicists and the general public. The need for a strong regulatory framework is crucial to ensure that this technology is used responsibly.

e. Future prospects

As the technology continues to evolve, we are likely to see the emergence of new variants of the CRISPR system that will further improve its precision and efficiency. Research is also underway to extend its use beyond gene editing to other fields such as gene therapy and even synthetic biology.

Challenges and ethical considerations

The CRISPR-Cas9 system, which makes it possible to edit the genome with unprecedented precision, has aroused considerable interest in the fields of biology, medicine and agriculture. However, its use raises complex ethical and regulatory challenges that require careful attention.

Ethical Challenges

Human genetic modification: One of the main ethical challenges is linked to the genetic modification of human embryos. The implications of such a practice are vast, including the possibility of creating "designer babies" or introducing hereditary modifications that could affect future generations. This raises questions about human identity, equal access to advanced technologies and unforeseen consequences for human biodiversity.

Informed consent: In research involving CRISPR-Cas9, informed consent becomes a crucial issue. Research participants must be fully informed of the potential risks associated with genome editing, as well as the ethical implications of their contributions.

Social justice: Unequal access to CRISPR technologies could exacerbate existing social inequalities. Developed countries could benefit more from these technological advances, while developing countries could lag behind, creating an even greater gap between different populations.

Regulatory Challenges

Inadequate regulatory framework: Currently, there is a lack of international consensus regarding the regulation of CRISPR-Cas9 use. Laws vary considerably from country to country, complicating cross-border research and leading to potential abuses in less stringent jurisdictions.

Monitoring and liability: The question of who is liable in the event of adverse effects or accidents linked to the use of CRISPR is also of concern. Clear mechanisms for monitoring CRISPR applications are essential to ensure that researchers and practitioners act responsibly.

Ongoing ethical assessment: It is imperative that ethics committees and regulatory bodies continue to regularly assess the ethical and social implications of CRISPR-Cas9 as the technology evolves. This includes the development of clear guidelines for its use in various contexts.

3. Clinical and ethical applications of gene therapy

Gene therapy is an innovative approach to treating or preventing disease by modifying an individual's genes. This method has attracted growing interest in the medical field, as it offers the possibility of treating hereditary genetic diseases, cancers and other serious conditions. However, clinical applications of gene therapy also raise complex ethical issues.

Clinical applications of gene therapy

Gene therapy studies focus mainly on two approaches: the insertion of healthy genes to replace defective ones, and the use of techniques such as CRISPR to directly modify existing genes. Clinical trials have been carried out to treat various conditions such as :

- **Monogenic diseases**: These diseases are caused by a mutation in a single gene. Gene therapy can potentially correct these mutations, as in the case of spinal muscular atrophy or certain forms of muscular dystrophy.

- **Cancers**: Gene therapy is used to introduce genes that can stimulate the immune system to attack cancer cells, or to make tumor cells more sensitive to treatment.

- **Viral diseases**: Research is underway into the use of gene therapy to treat chronic viral infections, such as HIV.

Ethical practices related to gene therapy: The rise of gene therapy raises several ethical issues:

- **Safety and efficacy**: The risks associated with genetic modification, including off-target effects and immune reactions, must be carefully assessed before any clinical application.

- **Informed consent**: Patients must be fully informed of potential risks and benefits before accepting gene therapy treatment.

- **Equity of access**: There are concerns about unequal access to advanced treatments, which could exacerbate health inequalities.

- **Germline vs. somatic modification**: The distinction between somatic genetic modification (which affects only the patient) and germline modification (which can be passed on to future generations) raises profound ethical questions about potential eugenics and the right to genetic integrity.

- **Regulation and surveillance**: public policies must evolve to provide a framework for these new technologies, while protecting the rights of individuals and guaranteeing responsible research.

Practical work: Gene therapy of inflammatory diseases

Gene therapy is an innovative approach to treating or preventing disease by modifying an individual's genes. In the context of inflammatory diseases, this technique offers promising potential for targeting the underlying mechanisms of inflammation and improving patients' quality of life. Here's a practical assignment you can give students on this topic.

Objective: Understand the principles of gene therapy and its application in the treatment of inflammatory diseases.

Instructions :

- **Bibliographic Research:** Students are expected to conduct in-depth research on gene therapy, focusing specifically on its use in inflammatory diseases such as rheumatoid arthritis, Crohn's disease and ulcerative colitis.

  They must identify at least three case studies where gene therapy has been successfully applied or shown significant potential.

- **Report Writing:** Write a 2000-word report that includes:

  - An introduction to gene therapy and inflammatory diseases.
  - A detailed explanation of the mechanisms of action of gene therapy.
  - A critical analysis of selected case studies, including results achieved and challenges encountered.
  - A discussion on the future of gene therapy in the treatment of inflammatory diseases.

- **Presentation:** Prepare a 10-minute PowerPoint presentation summarizing the key points of the report. The presentation should include:

  - Graphics or images illustrating the concepts discussed.
  - Time for questions and answers at the end.

- **Personal Reflection:** Include a section in the report where each student reflects on the potential impact of gene therapy on their understanding of modern medical treatments and their ethics.

- **Assessment :** Students will be assessed on :
  - The depth and relevance of their research (30%).
  - Clarity and organization of the written report (30%).
  - Effectiveness and commitment during the presentation (20%).
  - Personal reflection and critical analysis (20%).

Chapter 4: Nanomedicine

I. Design and application of nanomaterials in medicine

Nanomedicine is an emerging field of medicine that uses nanoscale technologies for the diagnosis, treatment and prevention of disease. Nanomedicine is based on the principles of nanotechnology, which is the study and application of structures, devices and systems smaller than 100 nanometers. At this scale, the physical and chemical properties of materials can differ considerably from those observed at larger scales, opening up new possibilities for medical intervention.

Nanomedicine applications

1. **Diagnosis**:

Nanomaterials, with their unique properties such as large specific surface area, enhanced chemical reactivity and special optical characteristics, offer significant advantages in early disease diagnosis, tissue visualization and drug targeting.

Applications of Nanomaterials in Medical Diagnostics

- **Medical imaging**: Nanoparticles are used as contrast agents in various medical imaging techniques, including MRI (magnetic resonance imaging) and PET (positron emission tomography). For example, gold nanoparticles can enhance contrast in MRI thanks to their ability to interact with magnetic fields.

- **Biomarkers**: Nanomaterials can be functionalized to bind specifically to certain disease-associated biomarkers. This enables more precise and sensitive detection of diseases such as cancer. Studies show that sensors based on carbon nanotubes or silver nanoparticles can detect very low concentrations of tumor biomarkers.

- **Targeted Delivery Systems**: In diagnosis and treatment, nanomaterials can be used to deliver therapeutic agents directly to diseased cells, while enabling real-time monitoring via imaging. This not only improves treatment efficacy but also reduces side effects.

- **Rapid diagnostic tests**: Nanomaterial-based devices are enabling the development of rapid diagnostic tests for various infections or medical conditions. For example, tests using gold nanoparticles to rapidly detect the presence of antigens or antibodies in a biological sample have become popular.

- **Nanosensors**: These devices exploit the unique electronic and optical properties of nanomaterials to detect changes in the biological environment that could indicate disease. They are capable of providing a rapid and sensitive response to chemical variations associated with pathologies.

2. Targeted therapy:

Targeted therapy is an innovative approach to the treatment of diseases such as cancer. Unlike traditional treatments that affect both healthy and diseased cells, targeted therapy specifically targets cancer cells, minimizing side effects and improving treatment efficacy. The integration of nanomaterials into this approach has opened up new avenues for the development of more effective drugs.

1. Nanomaterials in medicine

Nanomaterials, defined as materials with at least one dimension in the nanometric range (1 to 100 nm), have unique properties that make them particularly suitable for use in medicine. Their small size enables them to interact with biomolecules at a fundamental level, facilitating targeted drug delivery. For example, nanoparticles can be designed to bind specifically to receptors present on tumor cells, enabling localized drug release directly into the tumor.

2. Mechanisms of action: The mechanisms by which nanomaterials exert their therapeutic effect are varied. They can act in several ways:

- **Targeted delivery**: nanoparticles can be modified to carry chemotherapeutic agents or therapeutic genes to specific cells.
- **Medical imaging**: nanomaterials are also used as contrast agents in medical imaging, enabling early and accurate detection of tumors.
- **Combination therapies**: By integrating several types of treatment (such as chemotherapy and immunotherapy) in a single nanoparticle system, it is possible to increase the overall efficacy of treatment.

3. Clinical applications: Numerous clinical studies have been carried out to assess the efficacy of targeted therapies using nanomaterials. For example, some lipid nanoparticle formulations have shown an enhanced ability to effectively deliver paclitaxel (a chemotherapeutic agent) while reducing its systemic side effects.

4. Challenges and prospects: Despite their potential advantages, the use of nanomaterials in targeted therapy also presents a number of challenges. Biocompatibility, potential toxicity and in vivo stability are all concerns that need to be taken into account when developing these therapeutic systems. In addition, clear regulatory protocols are essential to ensure the safety and efficacy of these new approaches.

3. Vaccines and immunological therapies with nanomaterial applications

Vaccines and immunotherapies represent significant advances in preventive and therapeutic medicine. Their development is based on an in-depth understanding of the immune system, as well as on technological innovation, notably the use of nanomaterials.

Vaccines and Immunological Therapies: Vaccines work by stimulating the immune system to recognize and fight specific pathogens. They often contain antigens derived from viruses or bacteria, which are administered to induce an immune response without causing disease. Immunological therapies, meanwhile, include a wide range of approaches aimed at modulating the immune response to treat various diseases, including cancers.

Mechanisms of action: Vaccines fall into several categories:

- **Live attenuated vaccines**: Contain live but weakened pathogens.
- **Inactivated vaccines**: composed of killed pathogens.
- **Subunit vaccines**: Contain only specific parts of the pathogen (antigens).
- **DNA or RNA vaccines**: Use genetic material to induce an immune response.

Immunological therapies include :

- **Monoclonal antibody immunotherapy**: Use of antibodies specifically targeting tumor cells.
- **Cell therapy**: Transplantation of immune cells modified to improve their ability to fight cancer.

Nanomaterial applications: The integration of nanomaterials in the development of vaccines and immunotherapies has opened up promising new avenues. Nanomaterials can enhance antigen delivery, increase the efficacy of adjuvants (substances that boost the immune response) and enable controlled drug release.

Types of Nanomaterials Used

- **Lipid nanoparticles**: used to encapsulate antigens and facilitate their absorption by antigen-presenting cells.
- **Polymeric nanoparticles**: offer a flexible platform for targeted delivery of therapeutic agents.
- **Carbon nanotubes**: have unique properties that can be exploited to transport drugs or as vectors in vaccines.

Benefits

- **Enhanced immunogenicity**: nanoparticles can present antigens in a way that stimulates the immune system more effectively.
- **Targeted delivery**: Reduces side effects by concentrating treatment on target cells.
- **Controlled release**: Ensures that the drug is released at the right time and at the right place in the body.

4. Tissue engineering:

Tissue engineering is an interdisciplinary field that combines principles from biology, engineering, medicine and materials science to develop biological substitutes capable of restoring, maintaining or improving the function of damaged tissues or organs. This field of study emerged in the 1980s and has grown exponentially thanks to technological advances and a better understanding of the underlying biological mechanisms.

Fundamental concepts

- **Biomaterials**: Biomaterials are essential in tissue engineering. They must be biocompatible, i.e. they must not provoke an undesirable immune response when implanted in the body. Biomaterials can be natural (such as collagen) or synthetic (such as biodegradable polymers).

- **Stem cells**: Stem cells play a crucial role in tissue engineering, as they have the ability to differentiate into the various cell types required for tissue regeneration. Research into embryonic and adult stem cells has opened up new avenues for cell therapy.

- **Scaffolds**: Scaffolds are three-dimensional structures that support cell growth and new tissue formation. They must have an appropriate architecture to promote cell adhesion, proliferation and differentiation.

- **Growth factors**: These proteins regulate various cellular processes, including proliferation, migration and differentiation of cells. Targeted application of growth factors can improve the efficacy of tissue engineering treatments.

- **Clinical applications**: Tissue engineering has a number of promising clinical applications, including the treatment of skin injuries, cardiovascular disease, orthopedic disorders and even some approaches to degenerative diseases such as diabetes.

Current practices: Current tissue engineering practices include:

- **Cell culture**: In vitro culture enables us to study cell behavior in a controlled environment prior to clinical application.

- **3D printing**: This technology enables the creation of complex structures that mimic the natural architecture of human tissue.

- **Combination therapies**: Integrating pharmacological approaches with tissue engineering to optimize therapeutic outcomes.

- **Clinical trials**: Many tissue engineering projects go through clinical trials to assess their safety and efficacy before being approved for general use.

5. Biosensors

Biosensors, which are analytical devices capable of detecting biological substances, have undergone a significant evolution thanks to the integration of nanomaterials. Due to their unique properties at the nanoscale, nanomaterials offer considerable advantages for improving the sensitivity and specificity of biosensors. In-depth studies on biosensors using nanomaterials focus on several key aspects: sensor design, detection mechanisms, and practical applications in various fields such as health, the environment and agriculture.

1. Nanomaterial properties: Nanomaterials have a large specific surface area and improved optical, electrical and catalytic properties. These characteristics enable biosensors to achieve enhanced sensitivity when detecting biomolecules such as proteins, nucleic acids or metabolites.

2. Biosensor design: The design of biosensors incorporating nanomaterials often involves the use of gold nanoparticles, graphene or carbon nanotubes. These materials can be used as transducers to convert the biological signal into a measurable signal. For example, gold nanoparticles can amplify the electrochemical signal when reacting with a specific target.

3. Detection mechanisms: Detection mechanisms in nanomaterial-based biosensors mainly include electrochemical and optical detection. In the case of electrochemical detection, nanomaterials facilitate electron transfer between the sensor and the biological target. As for optical methods, the plasmonic properties of nanoparticles can be exploited to detect changes in light intensity in response to biomolecule binding.

4. Practical applications: The practical applications of biosensors using nanomaterials are vast:

- **Health**: Early detection of disease through blood analysis.
- **Environment**: Monitoring pollutants in water or air.
- **Agriculture**: Monitoring water stress in plants or rapid detection of pathogens.

6. **Future prospects:** The future of nanomaterial-based biosensors looks promising, with continued advances in nanotechnology and their integration with other emerging technologies such as artificial intelligence to further enhance their effectiveness and reach.

II. Drug targeting

Nanomedicine is an emerging field that uses nanoscale systems to improve the diagnosis, treatment and prevention of disease. Nanomedicine drug targeting is an innovative approach that aims to deliver therapeutic agents directly to diseased cells or tissues while minimizing side effects on healthy cells. This method is based on several fundamental principles, including nanoparticle design, surface functionalization and the use of biological vectors.

1. Nanoparticle design

Nanoparticles, defined as particles between 1 and 100 nanometers in size, are at the heart of much research due to their unique properties, which differ considerably from those of bulk materials. These particular properties include high specific surface area, enhanced chemical reactivity, and distinct optical, electrical and magnetic behaviors. In-depth studies on nanoparticles encompass various fields such as chemistry, physics, biology and engineering.

Nanoparticle design: The design of nanoparticles involves several methods which can be classified into two main categories: top-down and bottom-up.

- **Top-Down Methods**: These techniques start with a larger material which is progressively reduced to the nanoscale. This may involve mechanical processes such as grinding or machining, as well as chemical techniques such as laser erosion or lithography.

- **Bottom-Up methods**: In contrast to top-down methods, these techniques build nanoparticles from individual atoms or molecules. This can include processes such as chemical precipitation, self-assembly and sol-gel synthesis.

Nanoparticle applications: Nanoparticles have found applications in various fields:

- **Medicine**: used for drug targeting, medical imaging and cancer treatment.
- **Electronics**: Used in the manufacture of miniaturized electronic devices.
- **Environment**: Used for wastewater treatment and pollutant detection.
- **Advanced materials**: Incorporated into composites to improve their mechanical and thermal properties.

Nanoparticle characterization: Characterization is essential for understanding the physical and chemical properties of nanoparticles. Commonly used techniques include:

- **Transmission electron microscopy (TEM)**: Used to observe the internal structure of nanoparticles.

- **X-ray diffraction (XRD)**: Used to determine the crystalline phases present in samples.
- **Infrared (IR) spectroscopy**: Provides information on the functional groups present on the surface of nanoparticles.

Ethical and environmental challenges: The growing use of nanoparticles also raises a number of ethical and environmental concerns. Potential effects on human health and the environment need to be carefully assessed before widespread use.

2. Surface functionalization

Surface functionalization is a crucial area in the development of drug delivery systems. It involves the chemical or physical modification of material surfaces to enhance their interaction with biomolecules, which is essential for precise drug targeting. This approach aims to increase therapeutic efficacy while reducing side effects.

a. **Fundamental concepts:** Surface functionalization can be achieved by several methods, including surface chemistry, molecular self-assembly and the use of polymers. These techniques make it possible to introduce specific functional groups onto the surface of a material, which can influence its biological properties. For example, nanoparticles can be modified to display specific ligands that bind to particular cellular receptors, facilitating targeted drug delivery.
b. **Drug targeting applications:** Functionalized drug delivery systems are used in a variety of clinical contexts, notably in cancer treatment, where they can specifically target tumor cells while sparing healthy tissue. Liposomes and polymeric nanoparticles are often used as vectors to carry therapeutic agents. Functionalization not only enhances drug bioavailability, but also optimizes its controlled release.
c. **Characterization techniques:** To assess the effectiveness of functionalization, a variety of analytical techniques are employed. Infrared spectroscopy (FTIR), scanning electron microscopy (SEM) and chromatography are commonly used to characterize surface modifications and to analyze the interaction between the carrier and the drug.
d. **Challenges and future prospects:** Despite significant advances in this field, a number of challenges remain. The homogeneity of functionalization, the long-term stability of the systems developed

and their in vivo behavior remain subjects of intense research. In addition, it is crucial to assess the potential toxicity associated with functionalized materials.

As our understanding of biomolecular interactions deepens, we are likely to see the emergence of innovative new strategies to further improve drug targeting via surface functionalization.

3. Biological vectors

The use of biological vectors for drug targeting is a rapidly expanding field of research that combines molecular biology, pharmacology and biomedical engineering. Biological vectors, such as liposomes, nanoparticles and modified viruses, are designed to transport therapeutic agents directly to target cells while minimizing side effects on healthy tissue.

1. Basic concepts of biological vectors: Biological vectors are often used to enhance the bioavailability and specificity of drugs. For example, liposomes can encapsulate hydrophobic drugs and facilitate their transport in the body. In addition, these systems can be surface-modified to specifically target certain cells or tissues via specific ligands that bind to cellular receptors.

2. Types of biological vectors

- **Liposomes**: These are spherical vesicles composed of a lipid bilayer that can encapsulate various types of drug. They are widely used to improve drug solubility and stability.

- **Nanoparticles**: These nano-scale structures can be manufactured from a variety of materials (polymers, metals) and, thanks to their small size, enable precise targeting.

- **Viral vectors**: Modified viruses can be used to deliver genetic material or therapeutic proteins directly into target cells. This approach is particularly promising in the treatment of genetic diseases and certain cancers.

3. Clinical applications: Biological vectors have found applications in a number of therapeutic fields:

- **Oncology**: Targeted nanoparticles can deliver chemotherapeutic agents directly to tumors, reducing systemic toxicity.

- **Gene therapy**: the use of viral vectors to introduce corrective genes into defective cells in patients suffering from hereditary diseases.

- **Vaccines**: Biological vectors also play a crucial role in the development of innovative vaccines, particularly those based on messenger RNA.

4. Challenges and future prospects: Despite their potential advantages, the use of biological vectors presents several challenges:

- **Immunogenicity**: Some vectors may induce an undesirable immune response that could reduce their efficacy.

- **Targeting control**: Ensuring that the drug reaches only the target cells without affecting healthy cells remains a major challenge.

Future research will focus on optimizing these systems to improve their efficacy while reducing their side effects.

4. Clinical evaluation and challenges

Drug targeting is a therapeutic approach that aims to deliver pharmacological agents directly to diseased cells or tissues while minimizing the impact on healthy cells. This strategy is particularly relevant in the treatment of cancer, where traditional drugs can cause serious side effects due to their non-specific action. In-depth studies on drug targeting focus on several key aspects, including molecule design, mechanisms of action, delivery systems and clinical evaluation.

- **Molecule design:** Targeted drug design relies on understanding disease-specific biomarkers. Researchers often use molecular biology to identify these targets, enabling the development of more effective therapies. For example, monoclonal antibodies are designed to bind to specific antigens present on tumor cells. This enables selective destruction of cancer cells while sparing healthy cells.
- **Mechanisms of action:** The mechanisms of action of targeted drugs can vary considerably. Some act by directly inhibiting the cell signaling that promotes tumor growth, while others may induce an immune response against cancer cells. Research continues to explore these mechanisms in order to improve efficacy and reduce resistance to treatment.

- **Delivery systems:** Delivery systems play a crucial role in the success of drug targeting. Technologies such as nanoparticles and liposomes are used to encapsulate drugs and facilitate their transport to the target site. These systems also enable precise control of drug release, which can improve efficacy while reducing side effects.
- **Clinical evaluation:** Clinical evaluation of targeted therapies involves several phases of rigorous clinical trials to determine their safety and efficacy. Studies must demonstrate not only that the drug effectively targets its target, but also that it actually improves clinical outcomes compared with standard treatments.

III. using nanotechnologies for medical imaging

Nanotechnologies, which involve the manipulation of matter on a nanometric scale (1 to 100 nanometers), have aroused growing interest in the field of medical imaging. These technologies make it possible to improve the precision and efficiency of imaging techniques, while opening up new avenues for the diagnosis and treatment of disease.

Nanotechnology applications in medical imaging

- **Nanoparticles as contrast agents**: Nanoparticles can be used as contrast agents in various imaging modalities, including MRI (magnetic resonance imaging), PET (positron emission tomography) and ultrasound. For example, gold nanoparticles and iron nanoparticles are often used to enhance the contrast of MRI images, enabling better visualization of tissues and organs.

- **Targeted imaging**: Nanotechnologies also enable targeted imaging, where contrast agents are designed to bind specifically to certain cells or biomarkers. This not only improves early detection of disease, but also enables more accurate assessment of response to treatment.

- **Combination therapies**: The integration of nanotechnologies with imaging techniques enables the development of combination therapies, where imaging is used to guide targeted treatments. For example, nanoparticles can be designed to deliver drugs while providing real-time visualization of the therapeutic process.

- **Molecular imaging**: advances in nanotechnology have enabled the development of molecular imaging tools that can detect changes at the cellular and molecular level. This is particularly useful for monitoring cancer and other chronic diseases.

- **Ethical and regulatory challenges**: Although the potential benefits are considerable, there are also challenges associated with the use of nanotechnologies in medical imaging, particularly with regard to safety, ethics and regulation. The potential toxicity of nanoparticles and their behavior in the human body require extensive research before widespread clinical use.

Practical work on the rehabilitation of ankle sprains

Rehabilitation of ankle sprains is a crucial topic in the field of physiotherapy and sports medicine. Ankle sprains are common injuries, often caused by a sudden twist or movement that stretches or tears the ligaments that stabilize the joint. Rehabilitation is essential to restore function, reduce pain and prevent recurrence.

Objective: Understand the fundamental principles of ankle sprain rehabilitation and apply this knowledge through practical exercises.

1. Initial assessment

- **Aim: To** learn how to assess an ankle sprain.
- **Activity:** Have students perform a physical assessment on a partner simulating a sprain (using criteria such as swelling, pain, range of motion).

2. Acute phase (Days 1-3)

- **Goal:** Understand the principles of RICE (Rest, Ice, Compression, Elevation).
- **Activity:** Simulate the initial treatment of a sprain by applying cold and elevating the injured limb.

3. Subacute phase (Days 4-14)

- **Goal:** Introduce light exercises to improve range of motion.
- **Activity:** Design an exercise program including gentle movements such as passive and active flexion/extension.

4. Rehabilitation phase (Weeks 2-6)

- **Purpose: To** strengthen the muscles around the ankle.
- **Activity:** Create an exercise circuit including :
    - Exercises with elastic bands to strengthen the peroneal muscles.
    - Balance exercises on one leg to improve proprioception.

5. Back to sport (Weeks 6+)

- **Goal:** Prepare the patient to return to sports activities.
- **Activity:** Develop a progressive training plan incorporating movements specific to the patient's sport, while monitoring for signs of pain or discomfort.

Conclusion

Students must be able not only to apply these techniques, but also to justify each step of the rehabilitation process based on the underlying anatomical and physiological principles.

Chapter 5: Generative medicine

Introduction

Regenerative medicine is an innovative field of biology and medicine that aims to repair, replace or regenerate damaged tissues and organs. It relies on the use of stem cells, biomaterials and other advanced techniques to restore normal physiological functions. This discipline is emerging as a response to the limitations of traditional treatments, particularly in the context of degenerative diseases, traumatic injuries and aging.

Foundations of Regenerative Medicine: Regenerative medicine is based on several key concepts:

- **Stem cells**: Stem cells are undifferentiated cells capable of transforming into various cell types. They play a crucial role in tissue repair, and are at the heart of regenerative medicine research.

- **Biomaterials**: These synthetic or natural materials are used to support cell growth and promote tissue regeneration. They can be designed to mimic the mechanical and biological properties of natural tissues.

- **Tissue engineering**: This approach combines cells, biomaterials and growth factors to create tissue structures that can be implanted in the human body.

- **Gene therapies**: Integrating specific genes into cells can improve their ability to repair themselves or develop into functional tissues.

- **Clinical applications**: Regenerative medicine has already demonstrated its potential in the treatment of various conditions such as heart disease, spinal cord injury, neurodegenerative disorders, and even some forms of cancer.

Future prospects: Technological advances continue to broaden the horizons of regenerative medicine. In-depth research into the biological mechanisms underlying regenerative processes is helping to optimize existing treatments and develop new ones. However, this field faces a number of ethical and regulatory challenges that require careful attention to ensure that these innovations are implemented safely and effectively.

I. Stem cells: sources and applications

Stem cells are undifferentiated cells capable of transforming into various cell types and multiplying indefinitely. Their in-depth study and application in regenerative medicine have attracted growing interest in recent decades, as they offer promising prospects for the treatment of various diseases and injuries.

Stem cell sources: Stem cells can be classified into several categories according to their origin:

1. Embryonic stem cells (ESC) :

Embryonic stem cells (ESCs) are pluripotent cells with the ability to differentiate into almost any cell type in the human body. They are derived from embryos at an early stage of development, generally from the blastocyst, a structure formed around five days after fertilization. The in-depth study and practices associated with ESCs encompass many fields, including cell biology, regenerative medicine, ethics and therapeutic applications.

Advanced Embryonic Stem Cell Studies

- **Biological characteristics**: ESCs are distinguished by their ability to self-renew indefinitely while retaining their pluripotency. This means they can give rise to all cell types, including neurons, cardiomyocytes and other specialized cells. This characteristic is essential for normal embryonic development and offers promising prospects for biomedical research.

- **Therapeutic applications**: ESCs are being studied for their potential in the treatment of various degenerative diseases such as Parkinson's disease, type 1 diabetes and spinal cord injury. By using ESCs to generate specific cells, it is possible to envisage regenerative therapies where damaged tissues can be repaired or replaced.

- **Culture techniques**: in vitro culture of ESCs requires specific conditions to maintain pluripotency and avoid premature differentiation. Techniques such as the use of growth factor-enriched media are essential to support their growth.

- **Ethics and regulations**: The use of ESCs raises important ethical questions concerning the destruction of human embryos to obtain these cells. Many countries have put in place strict regulations concerning ESC research in order to balance scientific potential with moral considerations.

- **Current research**: Recent research has focused on improving ESC derivation and culture methods, as well as exploring new ways of using these cells in the clinical setting. Studies are also investigating the use of technologies such as CRISPR-Cas9 to genetically modify these cells to enhance their therapeutic capabilities.

Practices associated with Embryonic Stem Cells: Practices surrounding the use of ESCs include:

- **Cell derivation**: Derivation involves the careful extraction of stem cells from embryos without compromising their integrity.
- **Controlled differentiation**: Researchers are working on protocols for controlled differentiation into specific cell lines.
- **Cell transplantation**: Once differentiated, these cells can be transplanted into a host organism to treat various pathologies.
- **Safety assessment**: Before any clinical application, it is crucial to assess the safety and efficacy of ESC-based treatments.

2. Adult stem cells :

Adult stem cells, also known as somatic stem cells, are undifferentiated cells found in various tissues of the adult body. Unlike embryonic stem cells, which originate in embryos and have the capacity to differentiate into any cell type, adult stem cells have a more limited capacity for differentiation. However, they play a crucial role in tissue regeneration and repair.

In-depth studies on adult stem cells

- **Origin and types**: Adult stem cells are found in many tissues, including bone marrow, peripheral blood, adipose tissue and certain organs such as the liver and brain. They can be classified into two broad categories: hematopoietic stem cells (which give rise to the various blood cells) and mesenchymal stem cells (which can differentiate into bone, cartilage and adipose tissue).

- **Regeneration mechanisms**: Adult stem cells are essential for maintaining tissue homeostasis. They are activated in response to injury or physiological stress to replace lost or damaged cells. For example, after muscle injury, satellite cells (a type of muscle stem cell) divide to repair muscle tissue.

- **Clinical applications**: Adult stem cell research has led to significant advances in regenerative medicine. Therapies based on hematopoietic stem cell transplants are already being used to treat certain blood diseases such as leukemia. In addition, studies are exploring their potential in repairing the heart after a heart attack, or in treating neurodegenerative diseases such as Parkinson's.

- **Ethical and technical challenges**: Although the use of adult stem cells is generally considered less controversial than that of embryonic cells, it nevertheless poses ethical challenges linked to their collection and manipulation. Moreover, their clinical efficacy can vary according to the age of the donor and the general condition of the tissue of origin.

- **Future prospects**: Research continues to explore how to improve the isolation and culture of adult stem cells to increase their therapeutic potential. Techniques such as cell reprogramming aim to transform these cells into the specific cell types needed to treat various pathologies.

3. Induced pluripotent stem cells (iPSCs) :

Induced pluripotent stem cells (iPSCs) represent a major advance in the field of cell biology and regenerative medicine. These cells are derived from adult somatic cells that have been reprogrammed to a pluripotent state, meaning they have the capacity to differentiate into almost any cell type in the human body. This reprogramming is generally achieved by introducing specific transcription factors, such as Oct4, Sox2, Klf4 and c-Myc, which play a crucial role in maintaining pluripotency.

In-depth studies of CSPi

- **Origin and discovery**: iPSCs were first discovered in 2006 by Shinya Yamanaka and colleagues. Their work demonstrated that it was possible to reprogram murine fibroblasts into pluripotent cells using a cocktail of four genetic factors. This discovery paved the way for intensive research into the potential applications of iPSCs in the treatment of degenerative diseases and injuries.

- **Reprogramming mechanisms**: Reprogramming somatic cells into iPSCs involves several complex mechanisms, including epigenetic modification and reorganization of the gene expression network. Researchers are studying these mechanisms to better understand how to control the reprogramming process and improve the efficacy and safety of iPSCs.

- **Medical applications**: iPSCs offer considerable potential for regenerative medicine, notably in the treatment of diseases such as diabetes, neurodegenerative diseases (like Alzheimer's and Parkinson's), and gene therapy. Using iPSCs, patient-specific cells can be generated to replace or repair damaged tissue.

- **Ethical and technical challenges**: Although promising, iPSCs also raise ethical concerns regarding their use, particularly with regard to the risk of tumor formation (teratomas) during cell transplantation. In addition, there are still technical challenges to overcome to ensure that these cells are safe and effective for clinical use.

- **Future research**: The future of iPSC studies looks promising with the emergence of new technologies such as CRISPR-Cas9 genome editing, which could further improve the safety and efficacy of iPSC-based treatments. Research continues to explore not only their therapeutic applications but also their potential use in disease models to better understand various human disorders.

Applications in regenerative medicine: Stem cell applications in regenerative medicine are varied and include:

1. **Treatment of degenerative diseases** :

Degenerative diseases, also known as chronic degenerative diseases, are a group of conditions that lead to the progressive degradation of cells, tissues or organs. These diseases can affect various systems of the human body and are often age-related, although they can also be influenced by genetic, environmental and lifestyle factors. Here is a non-exhaustive list of some of the most common degenerative diseases:

- **Alzheimer's disease**: A form of dementia that affects memory, thinking and behavior. It is characterized by the formation of amyloid plaques and neurofibrillary degeneration in the brain.

- **Parkinson's disease**: A neurodegenerative disorder that mainly affects movement. It manifests itself in tremors, muscular rigidity and balance disorders.

- **Multiple sclerosis**: An autoimmune disease in which the immune system attacks myelin, the protective layer of the nerves, resulting in a variety of neurological symptoms.

- **Age-related macular degeneration (AMD)**: An eye condition that causes progressive loss of central vision due to deterioration of the retina.

- **Osteoarthritis**: A degenerative joint disease that causes articular cartilage to wear away, leading to pain and stiffness.

- **Amyotrophic lateral sclerosis (ALS)**: A neurodegenerative disease that affects motor neurons in the brain and spinal cord, leading to progressive muscle weakness.

- **Huntington's chorea**: An inherited disorder caused by a progressive degeneration of neurons in certain regions of the brain, leading to involuntary movements and cognitive impairment.

- **Idiopathic pulmonary fibrosis**: a chronic lung disease characterized by progressive scarring of lung tissue, making breathing difficult.

- **Type 2 diabetes**: Although often considered a metabolic disorder, it can lead to various degenerative complications such as cardiovascular disease and neuropathy.

- **Osteoporosis**: A condition characterized by a decrease in bone density and an increased risk of fractures.

Treatment of degenerative diseases in regenerative medicine

Regenerative medicine is an innovative field that aims to repair, replace or regenerate damaged cells, tissues or organs. Degenerative diseases, such as Alzheimer's, Parkinson's and degenerative spinal disorders, represent a major challenge to global public health. These conditions are often characterized by the progressive degradation of cells and tissues, leading to significant loss of function.

Approaches to Regenerative Medicine

a) **Stem cells**: Stem cells have the potential to differentiate into various cell types. Their use in the treatment of degenerative diseases relies on their ability to replace lost or damaged cells. For example, research into neural stem cells shows promising potential in the treatment of neurodegenerative diseases.

b) **Gene therapy**: Gene therapy involves introducing, eliminating or modifying genetic material within a patient's cells to treat a disease. In the context of degenerative diseases, this approach can correct the genetic mutations responsible for certain conditions.

c) **Tissue engineering**: This technique combines stem cells with biomaterials to create artificial tissues that can be implanted in the body to restore lost function. Studies have shown that tissue engineering could be used to treat spinal cord injuries and other traumatic injuries.

d) **Growth factors**: The use of growth factors to stimulate cell regeneration is also a promising avenue. These proteins can encourage cell proliferation and promote tissue repair in various degenerative pathologies.

e) **Nanotechnology**: The application of nanotechnology in regenerative medicine enables targeted drug delivery and better visualization of biological processes at the cellular level. This could improve the effectiveness of treatments for degenerative diseases.

Challenges and prospects: Despite these promising advances, several challenges remain in the field of regenerative medicine for the treatment of degenerative diseases:

- **Ethics**: The use of stem cells raises ethical questions about their origin.
- **Safety**: The risks associated with gene therapy and tissue implants must be carefully assessed.
- **Regulations**: The regulatory framework surrounding new therapies must evolve to guarantee their safety and efficacy.
- **Cost**: The development and clinical application of these technologies can be costly, limiting their accessibility.

2. Restorative medicine :

Restorative medicine, also known as regenerative medicine, is an innovative field of medicine that aims to repair or replace damaged tissues and organs. This field of study draws on advances in cell biology, tissue engineering and gene therapy to develop treatments capable of restoring the normal function of tissues affected by disease, injury or aging.

Key concepts

- **Cell and Tissue Biology**: Understanding stem cells is fundamental to restorative medicine. Stem cells are capable of differentiating into various cell types and can be used to regenerate damaged tissue. Research focuses on the isolation, culture and clinical application of these cells.

- **Tissue engineering**: This field combines the principles of engineering and biology to create biological substitutes that can mimic the natural structures of the human body. This includes the use of biomaterials to support cell growth and new tissue formation.

- **Gene therapy**: Gene therapy involves the introduction, removal or modification of genetic material within a patient's cells to treat a disease. This approach can be used to correct genetic defects that cause certain medical conditions.

- **Clinical applications**: Clinical applications of restorative medicine include the treatment of degenerative diseases such as Alzheimer's, spinal cord injury and cardiovascular disease, as well as orthopedics to repair damaged cartilage or bone.

- **Ethical and regulatory challenges**: Like any emerging field, restorative medicine raises ethical questions about the use of stem cells (particularly those derived from embryos), as well as regulatory concerns about the safety and efficacy of new therapies.

3. Gene therapies :

Gene therapies represent a significant advance in the field of regenerative medicine, offering potential solutions for treating genetic diseases, degenerative disorders and even certain forms of cancer. This therapeutic approach relies on the introduction, removal or modification of genetic material within a patient's cells to correct underlying genetic abnormalities or improve cellular function.

a) **Foundations of gene therapy**
Gene therapies can be divided into two main categories: somatic and germline. Somatic therapies aim to modify genes in an individual's somatic (non-reproductive) cells, while germline therapies involve modifications in germ cells (sperm and egg cells), which can have an impact on offspring.
The vectors used to deliver the genetic material are often derived from modified viruses, which have been engineered to be non-pathogenic yet have the ability to efficiently introduce the therapeutic gene into target cells. These include lentiviruses, adenoviruses and adeno-associated viruses (AAV).

a) **Clinical applications**
The clinical applications of gene therapies are vast. For example, they have shown promising potential in the treatment of hereditary diseases such as spinal muscular atrophy (SMA) and certain forms of muscular dystrophy. Clinical trials have demonstrated that the administration of corrective genes can significantly improve the quality of life of patients suffering from these conditions.
Gene therapy is also being explored for the treatment of cancer. By introducing genes that stimulate an immune response against tumor cells, or by inhibiting specific oncogenes, it is possible to increase the efficacy of traditional anti-cancer treatments.

b) **Challenges and ethical considerations**
Despite its promise, gene therapy raises a number of technical and ethical challenges. The risks associated with random insertion of genetic material can lead to undesirable effects such as activation of oncogenes or suppression of tumor suppressor genes. In addition, the ethical issues surrounding the manipulation of human genetic material are complex and require careful consideration of the long-term implications.

c) **Future prospects**
The future of gene therapy in regenerative medicine looks promising, thanks to technological advances such as CRISPR-Cas9, which enables precise genome editing. This opens the way to more targeted and potentially less risky treatments for various diseases.

4. **Organ transplantation**

Organ transplantation is a complex medical procedure involving the transfer of an organ from a donor to a recipient, with the aim of replacing a failing organ. In the context of regenerative medicine, this practice takes on an even more significant dimension, as it is part of an approach aimed not only at replacing organs, but also at restoring biological functions through tissue regeneration.

- **Historical background and development :** Organ transplantation has undergone major advances since the first successful transplants in the early 20th century. Advances in immunology, surgery and pharmacology have improved transplant success rates. The discovery of immunosuppressants has been particularly crucial in preventing transplant rejection by the recipient's immune system.
- **Regenerative medicine:** Regenerative medicine encompasses a variety of strategies aimed at repairing or replacing damaged tissues or organs. These include the use of stem cells, tissue bioengineering and gene therapy. These approaches aim to develop sustainable solutions for patients suffering from chronic or degenerative diseases.
- **Transplantation techniques:** Transplantation techniques can be classified into several categories:
  - **Allogeneic transplantation**: where the organ comes from a human donor.
  - **Autologous transplantation**: where the organ is taken from the same individual.
  - **Xenograft**: where the organ comes from a different species.

  Each of these methods presents its own challenges, particularly in terms of immune rejection and organ availability.
- **Ethical and social challenges:** Transplantation practices also raise important ethical issues, such as the commercialization of organs, informed consent of donors and equity of access to care. The shortage of available organs remains a major problem, prompting researchers to explore alternatives such as laboratory-grown organs.
- **Future prospects:** The future of organ transplantation as part of regenerative medicine looks promising, thanks to technological advances such as 3D organ printing and advanced cellular therapies. These innovations could potentially reduce reliance on donated human organs while improving clinical outcomes for patients.

Practical work on clinical trials in regenerative medicine

Introduction to Clinical Trials in Regenerative Medicine

Regenerative medicine is an innovative field that aims to repair, replace or regenerate damaged tissues and organs. Clinical trials play a crucial role in the development of new regenerative therapies, enabling the efficacy and safety of treatments to be assessed before they are brought to market. This practical work aims to explore the different stages of clinical trials, the challenges associated with regenerative medicine, and the importance of regulation and ethics in this field.

Practical work objectives

- **Understanding the Phases of Clinical Trials**: Students will study the different phases of clinical trials (Phase I, II, III and IV) and their respective importance in the development of treatments in regenerative medicine.

- **Analyzing Case Studies**: Students will be asked to choose a specific regenerative therapy (e.g. cell or gene therapies) and analyze a relevant clinical trial. They will be asked to examine methodology, results and ethical implications.

- **Assessing Ethical and Regulatory Challenges**: Students will be asked to discuss the ethical challenges associated with clinical trials in regenerative medicine, including informed consent, genetic manipulation and equitable access to treatments.

- **Report writing**: At the end of the practical work, each student will write a detailed report presenting his or her findings on the chosen clinical trial, including a discussion of its potential impact on medical practice.

- **Oral presentation**: Students will present their results in front of their peers to encourage an exchange of ideas and critical discussion on the subject.

Report structure: The report must include the following sections:

- **Introduction**
    - Overview of regenerative medicine.

- Importance of clinical trials.

- **Methodology of the chosen clinical trial**: Description of the trial (objective, target population, design).

- **Results**: Summary of results obtained.

- **Discussion**
    - Critical analysis of results.
    - Ethical and regulatory implications.

Conclusion

Final thoughts on the future of clinical trials in regenerative medicine.

II. Tissue imaging

Tissue imaging in regenerative medicine is a rapidly expanding field of research that combines advanced imaging techniques with therapeutic approaches aimed at repairing or replacing damaged tissue. This discipline relies on the ability to visualize and analyze tissue structures at different levels, from microscopic to macroscopic, to better understand the biological processes involved in tissue regeneration.

1. Foundations of tissue imaging

Tissue imaging uses a variety of imaging modalities, including MRI (magnetic resonance imaging), CT (computed tomography), ultrasound and light microscopy. Each of these techniques offers specific advantages for visualizing living tissue. For example, MRI is particularly useful for obtaining detailed images of soft tissues, while CT is often used to assess bone structures.

2. Applications in regenerative medicine

In regenerative medicine, tissue imaging plays a crucial role in monitoring treatments and evaluating the efficacy of cell and gene therapies. Researchers use these techniques to monitor tissue repair after injury or surgery, as well as to assess the viability and functionality of tissue grafts.

3. Advanced techniques

Advanced techniques such as fluorescence imaging and positron emission tomography (PET) are also being used to study metabolic processes within regenerative tissues. These methods provide dynamic information on cellular behavior and can help identify biomarkers associated with regeneration.

4. Challenges and future prospects

Despite the progress made, several challenges remain in the field of tissue imaging in regenerative medicine. One of the main challenges is to improve the spatial and temporal resolution of images while minimizing invasiveness for the patient. In addition, there is a growing need to integrate imaging data with other types of biological data to gain a holistic understanding of the regeneration process.

III. Cellular therapies for tissue repair.

Cell-based therapies for tissue repair represent a rapidly expanding field of research, incorporating innovative approaches aimed at restoring or replacing damaged tissue. These therapies rely on the use of living cells, often derived from a variety of sources such as stem cells, to promote tissue regeneration and treat degenerative diseases or injuries.

1. Types of Cell Therapy: Cell therapies can be classified into several categories:

- **Stem cells**: Embryonic and adult stem cells are at the heart of tissue regeneration research. They have the ability to differentiate into various cell types, making them ideal for replacing damaged cells in tissues such as cartilage, muscle or nerve tissue.

- **Gene therapy**: This approach combines cell therapy with genetic modification. Specific genes can be introduced into cells to correct genetic defects or improve their ability to repair tissue.

- **Exosome-based therapies**: Exosomes, small vesicles secreted by cells, play a crucial role in intercellular communication. They can carry proteins and messenger RNAs that promote tissue repair.

2. Mechanisms of action: The mechanisms by which these therapies act include :

- **Stimulation of angiogenesis**: the formation of new blood vessels is essential to supply the nutrients needed for tissue regeneration.

- **Modulation of the immune system**: certain stem cells have been shown to modulate the immune response, reducing inflammation and promoting an environment conducive to healing.

- **Growth factor secretion**: The cells used in these therapies secrete various growth factors that encourage cell proliferation and migration to the injured site.

3. Clinical applications: The clinical applications of cellular therapies are vast:

- **Orthopedics**: using stem cells to repair articular cartilage.

- **Cardiology**: Heart cell injections to improve cardiac function after a heart attack.

- **Neurology**: Research into the use of stem cells to treat spinal cord injuries and neurodegenerative diseases such as Alzheimer's.

4. Biological mechanisms

Cell therapy uses living cells to treat or prevent disease, focusing on the repair or replacement of damaged tissue. This process is based on an in-depth understanding of the biological mechanisms underlying tissue regeneration.

Biological Mechanisms in Cell Therapy

- **Stem cells**: Stem cells play a central role in cell therapy. They have the capacity to differentiate into various cell types and are essential for tissue development and repair. Research shows that mesenchymal stem cells (MSCs) can modulate immune responses and promote tissue regeneration through their ability to secrete trophic factors.
- **Cell signaling**: Signaling pathways, such as those involving cytokines and growth factors, are crucial in orchestrating tissue repair processes. For example, platelet-derived growth factor (PDGF) and epidermal growth factor (EGF) are involved in cell proliferation and migration to injured sites.
- **Tissue microenvironment**: The microenvironment plays a key role in the efficacy of cell-based therapies. Interactions between injected cells and host tissue can influence therapeutic outcome.

Studies show that remodeling the microenvironment can improve the integration of transplanted cells.

- **Tissue engineering**: Tissue engineering combines cells, biomaterials and biochemical factors to create functional tissue substitutes. This requires a thorough understanding of the mechanical and biological properties of the target tissue to optimize cell adhesion, proliferation and differentiation.
- **Clinical applications**: Clinical applications include the treatment of degenerative diseases such as osteoarthritis and cardiovascular disease, as well as acute and chronic injuries. Research continues to explore how to maximize therapeutic efficacy while minimizing the risks associated with cellular treatments.

Cell therapy administration techniques

Cell therapy involves the use of living cells to treat or prevent disease, and is particularly promising for the regeneration of damaged tissue. This approach relies on a number of delivery techniques designed to optimize the efficacy of transplanted cells while minimizing adverse effects.

Delivery Techniques in Cell Therapy

- **Direct injection**: One of the most common methods is to inject cells directly into the site of injury. This technique is often used to treat musculoskeletal injuries or degenerative diseases. Challenges include post-injection cell survival and homogeneous cell distribution in the target tissue.
- **Controlled-release systems**: These systems enable prolonged, controlled release of cells or associated growth factors. They may include hydrogels or other biomaterials that promote cell adhesion and migration to surrounding tissues.
- **Tissue engineering**: This approach combines cells with a three-dimensional scaffold that mimics the natural extracellular matrix of the target tissue. This not only provides structural support for the cells, but also enhances their integration into the host tissue.
- **Combined Gene Therapies**: In some cases, cells can be genetically modified prior to administration to enhance their therapeutic properties, such as the production of anti-inflammatory or pro-regenerative factors.
- **Systemic administration**: Although less targeted, this method uses the bloodstream to distribute cells throughout the body. It can

be useful in the treatment of systemic diseases where local intervention is not sufficient.

Challenges and prospects

Challenges associated with these techniques include cell survival after administration, immunogenicity, and functional integration within the host tissue. Ongoing research is needed to improve these methods, notably through the use of advanced biomaterials, optimization of injection protocols, and development of new tissue engineering strategies.

Practical work on Artificial Intelligence Modes Applied to Medical Imaging

Introduction

Artificial intelligence (AI) has revolutionized the field of medical imaging, offering powerful tools for the analysis and interpretation of visual data. This practical work aims to explore the various applications of AI in this field, focusing on techniques, algorithms and clinical outcomes.

Practical work objectives

- **Understanding AI Fundamentals**: Students should gain a basic understanding of artificial intelligence concepts, including machine learning, deep learning and their specific applications to medical imaging.

- **Exploring Medical Imaging Techniques**: Students will need to familiarize themselves with different imaging modalities (MRI, CT, ultrasound) and how they can be enhanced by AI algorithms.

- **Analyze Case Studies**: Students will be asked to examine several case studies where AI has been successfully applied to improve medical diagnosis or treatment.

- **Developing a Practical Project**: Using an available medical imaging dataset, each student will develop a simple machine learning model to classify or segment medical images.

- **Assess Ethical Implications**: Students will be asked to discuss the ethical implications of using AI in medicine, including data privacy and clinical liability.

Methodology

- **Bibliographical research**: Students will begin with an in-depth search of the academic literature to understand the theoretical foundations.
- **Hands-on workshops**: Practical sessions will be organized to enable students to manipulate AI tools and analyze real datasets.
- **Oral presentations**: Each student will present his or her results to the class, encouraging a critical exchange of ideas on their findings.

Conclusion

This practical work will enable students not only to acquire technical skills in AI applied to medical imaging, but also to develop critical thinking about its use in the medical field.

MODULE 2: MODERN SURGICAL TECHNIQUES

Introduction

The study of modern surgical techniques is a constantly evolving field, incorporating technological advances and innovative methods that are transforming surgical practice. Modern surgery is based on a thorough understanding of human anatomy and physiology, as well as the fundamental principles of medicine. Contemporary surgical techniques include not only traditional open procedures, but also less invasive approaches such as laparoscopy and robotics.

Advances in medical imaging, such as MRI and CT scans, have enabled surgeons to obtain precise visualization of the body's internal structures before performing an operation. This has led to more efficient surgical planning and a reduction in the risks associated with operations. In addition, the use of advanced surgical tools and technologies such as surgical navigation has improved the precision of interventions.

Continuing education is essential for healthcare professionals to familiarize themselves with these new techniques. Surgical residency programs now include modules on emerging technologies and evidence-based best practices. Ethics in modern surgery is also a crucial topic, as new technologies raise questions about informed consent and equity in access to care.

In addition, clinical research plays a fundamental role in assessing the efficacy and safety of new surgical procedures. Randomized clinical trials are often necessary to establish standardized protocols that guarantee the best possible outcome for patients.

In short, the study of modern surgical techniques involves a multidisciplinary approach that encompasses not only technical skills but also a thorough ethical and scientific understanding. This enables surgeons to offer optimal care while adapting to rapid developments in the medical field.

Chapter 6: Robot-assisted surgery

Introduction

Robot-assisted surgery (RAS) represents a significant advance in the medical field, combining robotic technologies with human surgical skills to improve patient outcomes. This innovative approach enables surgeons to perform complex procedures with greater precision, reduced post-operative pain and faster recovery times.

History and development

The use of robots in surgery began in the 1980s, but the technology really took off in the early 2000s with the introduction of the da Vinci system. This system enables surgeons to control miniaturized instruments remotely, providing a three-dimensional, enlarged view of the surgical field. Benefits include better tissue handling, less bleeding and reduced risk of infection.

Clinical applications

The applications of robot-assisted surgery are varied, and include procedures in urology, gynecology, cardiology and general surgery. In urology, for example, robot-assisted prostatectomy has become a standard procedure for the treatment of prostate cancer. Similarly, in gynecology, robot-assisted hysterectomy offers similar advantages in terms of rapid recovery and reduced complications.

Advantages and disadvantages : The main advantages of CAR include:

- **Greater precision**: Robots enable fine control of surgical instruments.
- **Less invasive**: Procedures can often be performed through smaller incisions.
- **Rapid recovery**: Patients generally benefit from a reduced hospital stay.

However, there are also potential drawbacks:

- **High cost**: Robotic equipment is expensive to acquire and maintain.
- **Learning curve**: Surgeons need specific training to master these systems.
- **Technical limitations**: Although robots are advanced, they do not completely replace human expertise.

Future prospects

The future of robot-assisted surgery looks bright with the continued integration of technological innovations such as artificial intelligence (AI) and augmented reality (AR). These technologies could further enhance surgical precision, enabling doctors to perform even more complex procedures with minimal risk to patients.

I. Principles of robotic surgery

Robotic surgery is a fast-growing specialty that combines technological advances in robotics with traditional surgical techniques. It offers significant advantages over conventional surgery, including greater precision, reduced invasiveness and faster recovery time for patients. The fundamentals of robotic surgery are based on several key elements: surgical robot technology, surgeon training, operating system ergonomics, and the integration of medical imaging.

1. Surgical robot technology

Robotic systems such as the Da Vinci Surgical System are designed to enable surgeons to perform complex procedures with great precision. These systems typically include a console where the surgeon controls the robotic instruments, as well as robotic arms that manipulate the surgical tools. The technology often employs high-definition 3D vision and magnification, enabling the surgeon to view the surgical field with exceptional clarity.

2. Surgeon training

Training is a crucial aspect in the adoption of robotic surgery. Training programs often include virtual simulations before surgeons begin operating on real patients. This enables them to acquire the skills needed to use robotic systems effectively, while minimizing the risks associated with learning in the field.

3. Operating system ergonomics

Ergonomics plays an essential role in the design of robotic systems. Designers strive to improve surgeon comfort during long surgical procedures, which can reduce fatigue and improve concentration. The user interface must also be intuitive to enable smooth, precise handling of the instruments.

4. Integration of medical imaging

The integration of advanced imaging technologies such as intra-operative ultrasound or MRI enables surgeons to obtain real-time information on the patient's anatomy during the operation. This improves not only the precision but also the overall safety of the surgical procedure.

5. The technical components of robotic surgery

Robotic surgery is a rapidly expanding field that combines advanced technology with the fundamental principles of surgical medicine. The technical components and underlying principles of this discipline are essential to understanding its operation and application in the clinical setting.

Technical Components for Robotic Surgery

- **Control systems**: At the heart of robotic surgery are sophisticated control systems that enable surgeons to operate with increased precision. These systems include advanced user interfaces, often based on touch screens, which enable the surgeon to manipulate robotic instruments with great finesse.

- **Robotic surgical instruments**: The instruments used in robotic surgery are designed to mimic the natural movements of human hands, while offering a superior range of motion. These instruments can include forceps, scalpels and other specialized tools that are often miniaturized to enable a less invasive procedure.

- **High-definition 3D vision**: Another key component is the vision system, which provides a high-definition, three-dimensional view of the surgical site. This gives the surgeon enhanced perception of depth and anatomical detail, which is crucial when performing delicate procedures.

- **Robotic platforms**: Robotic platforms themselves, such as the da Vinci system, incorporate several robotic arms controlled by the surgeon from a distance. These arms can be precisely positioned around the patient to perform a variety of surgical tasks.

- **Advanced software**: Software plays an essential role in the integration and operation of the various components of the robotic surgical system. It not only enables real-time control of the instruments, but also post-operative analysis and continuous improvement of surgical techniques.

Principles of Robotic Surgery

- **Minimizing invasiveness**: One of the main advantages of robotic surgery is its ability to perform less invasive procedures, reducing recovery time and lowering the risks associated with traditional surgery.

- **Improved precision**: Thanks to advanced technologies, procedures can be carried out with millimetric precision, which is particularly beneficial in complex operations such as those on the heart or brain.

- **Ergonomics for the surgeon**: The ergonomic design of robotic systems enables surgeons to operate in a comfortable position for long periods, reducing physical fatigue and improving concentration.

- **Training and Simulation**: Training in the use of robotic equipment often requires the use of advanced simulators that faithfully reproduce real operating conditions, enabling surgeons to acquire the necessary skills without risk to patients.

- **Interdisciplinary collaboration**: Robotic surgery often involves collaboration between various specialists such as biomedical engineers, computer scientists and physicians to ensure that all technical and clinical aspects are optimized for each procedure.

6. The challenges and ethical considerations involved in robotic surgery

Robotic surgery is a rapidly expanding discipline that uses robotic systems to assist surgeons during surgical procedures. While this technology offers significant advantages, such as increased precision, reduced post-operative pain and shorter recovery times, it also raises important ethical challenges that deserve particular attention.

- **Accuracy and liability:** One of the main ethical challenges associated with robotic surgery is the question of liability in the event of complications. When errors occur during robotic-assisted surgery, it can be difficult to determine whether the fault lies with the surgeon, the robotic system or a technical malfunction. This raises concerns about legal and professional liability, as well as the impact on patient trust in medical staff.
- **Informed consent:** Informed consent is a fundamental principle in medicine, requiring patients to be fully informed of the risks and benefits associated with any surgical procedure. In the context of robotic surgery, it

is crucial that patients understand not only how the robotic system works, but also the potential implications of such technology on their health. Practitioners need to ensure that patients are aware of the limitations of the technology and the skills required for its effective use.

- **Equity of access:** Another major ethical challenge concerns equity of access to advanced surgical technologies. Robotic surgery can be expensive and is not always available in all medical facilities, which can create inequalities in access to care. Policymakers need to think about how these technologies can be made available equitably, to avoid a gap between those who can afford these advanced treatments and those who can't.
- **Training and competence:** Proper training of surgeons using robotic systems is essential to ensure patient safety. However, there is debate about the level of competence required to operate these complex machines. Training programs need to be rigorous to ensure that only qualified professionals use these technologies, but this also raises questions about ongoing skills assessment throughout their careers.
- **Psychological impact on patients:** Finally, the increasing use of robots in surgery can have a psychological impact on patients. Some may experience heightened anxiety at the idea of being operated on by a machine rather than a human. It is therefore essential that healthcare professionals address these concerns with empathy, and provide adequate psychological support before and after the operation.

II. techniques

Telesurgery, an emerging branch of surgical medicine, uses advanced technologies to enable surgeons to perform procedures remotely. The practice relies on the integration of various technological tools, including robotics, telemedicine and real-time communication systems. In-depth studies of telesurgery techniques focus on several key aspects: the underlying technology, clinical applications, ethical and legal challenges, and the impact on surgical outcomes.

1. Underlying technology

Telesurgery, an emerging branch of computer-assisted surgery, relies on a complex set of technologies that enable surgeons to perform procedures remotely. This practice combines elements of robotics, real-time communication, advanced medical imaging and artificial intelligence to improve surgical outcomes while minimizing invasiveness.

Underlying Technologies

- **Surgical robotics**: Robotic systems such as the da Vinci system are at the heart of telesurgery. These robots enable precise manipulation of surgical instruments using articulated arms controlled by the surgeon via a console. Surgical robotics improve precision and reduce the surgeon's involuntary tremors.

- **Real-time communication**: Telesurgery requires a high-speed Internet connection to enable instantaneous data transmission between surgeon and patient. Secure communication protocols ensure that sensitive information is protected during surgery.

- **Advanced Medical Imaging**: The use of imaging tools such as ultrasound, computed tomography (CT) and magnetic resonance imaging (MRI) is essential to provide the surgeon with a detailed view of the patient's anatomy before and during the operation.

- **Artificial Intelligence (AI)**: AI is playing an increasing role in telesurgery, particularly in the analysis of preoperative and intraoperative data to aid surgical decision-making. Algorithms can also be used to predict potential complications based on the patient's medical history.

- **Haptic Control Systems**: These systems provide tactile feedback to the surgeon when using robotic instruments, enabling a more natural feel during remote surgical procedures.

Clinical practice: Clinical applications of telesurgery are developing rapidly in fields such as urological, gynecological, orthopedic and thoracic surgery. Studies show that clinical outcomes can be comparable to those of traditional surgical procedures, with additional benefits such as reduced hospitalization time and faster recovery for patients.

Ethical and technical challenges: Despite its potential advantages, telesurgery also raises a number of ethical and technical challenges. Questions relating to liability in the event of remote surgical complications need to be addressed. In addition, there are concerns about unequal access to the necessary technologies in different geographical regions.

2. Clinical applications

Telesurgery, an emerging branch of computer-assisted surgery, uses advanced technologies to enable surgeons to perform procedures remotely. This approach relies on the integration of several disciplines, including robotics, real-time communication systems and imaging technologies. In-depth studies on clinical applications of telesurgery focus on its potential benefits, its technical and ethical challenges, and its impact on surgical outcomes.

- **Benefits of telesurgery:** One of the key benefits of telesurgery is its ability to overcome geographical barriers. This enables patients in remote or underserved areas to access specialized care without having to travel to a medical center. In addition, telesurgery can reduce waiting times for certain surgical procedures, which can improve overall patient outcomes.
- **Techniques used :** Telesurgery techniques include the use of surgical robots that can be controlled by a remote surgeon. These systems are often equipped with high-definition cameras and miniaturized instruments, enabling greater precision during surgery. For example, the da Vinci system is widely used in various types of surgery, including urological and gynecological surgery.
- **Technical challenges:** Despite its advantages, telesurgery also presents a number of technical challenges. Communication latency can be a problem in delicate procedures, where every movement needs to be precisely synchronized. In addition, there are concerns about data security and patient privacy when information is transmitted via the Internet.
- **Ethical considerations:** Ethical considerations surrounding telesurgery include informed patient consent and the potential impact on the doctor-patient relationship. Patients must be informed that their procedure could be performed by a surgeon located at a distance, and understand the associated implications.

3. Ethical and legal challenges

Telesurgery, which refers to the use of technology to perform surgery at a distance, raises a multitude of ethical and legal challenges. These challenges are of crucial importance in today's context, where technological advances are transforming the medical landscape.

a. Ethical Challenges

The ethical challenges associated with telesurgery include issues of informed consent, medical liability, and equity of access to care. Informed consent is a fundamental principle in medicine, requiring patients to be fully informed of the risks and benefits of a procedure before consenting to it. In the context of telesurgery, it can be difficult for patients to fully understand the implications of a procedure carried out remotely, particularly in terms of quality of care and interaction with the surgeon. Medical liability is another tricky subject. In the event of a complication or error during a surgical procedure performed remotely, it can be difficult to determine who is liable: the surgeon, the hospital or the manufacturer of the equipment used. This raises questions about regulation and the need for a clear legal framework to protect both patients and healthcare professionals.

Finally, equity of access to care is a major issue. Telesurgery could exacerbate existing inequalities if certain populations do not have access to the necessary technologies, or if they do not benefit from the same level of technical competence in their care providers.

b. Legal challenges

From a legal point of view, a number of questions arise concerning the regulation of remote surgical practices. Laws vary considerably from country to country when it comes to medical practice, and this further complicates the situation when procedures are carried out across national borders. Practitioners have to navigate a complex legal landscape that can include laws on telemedicine, personal data protection (particularly with the RGPD in Europe), as well as specific professional standards.

Another important legal challenge is that related to health insurance and financial coverage for surgeries performed via telesurgery. Insurance companies may have different policies regarding reimbursement for these types of procedures, which may influence their adoption by medical establishments.

4. Impact on surgical results

Telesurgery, an emerging branch of computer-assisted surgery, uses advanced technologies to enable surgeons to perform procedures remotely. The practice relies on sophisticated communication systems that enable real-time transmission of images and data between the surgeon and the patient, often in a different location. The impact of telesurgery on medical training is significant and multidimensional.

a. **Evolving surgical skills:** Telesurgery training requires an adaptation of traditional skills. Surgeons must not only master conventional surgical techniques, but also become familiar with the use of advanced technological equipment. This includes handling surgical robots, interpreting images in real time, and managing the computer systems that underpin these procedures. Training programs must therefore incorporate these new skills to effectively prepare future practitioners.

b. **Simulation and virtual learning:** Simulation technologies play a crucial role in learning telesurgery techniques. Simulators enable medical students and residents to practice safely on virtual models before operating on real patients. These simulated environments provide a platform for developing both the technical skills and decision-making abilities required for remote surgery.
c. **Interdisciplinary collaboration:** Telesurgery also encourages a collaborative approach between different medical and technological disciplines. Training courses should include not only surgeons, but also biomedical engineers, IT specialists and other professionals involved in the development and application of surgical technologies. This collaboration enriches the educational process and enables technological innovations to be better integrated into clinical practice.
d. **Ethical and legal challenges:** The integration of telesurgery also raises ethical and legal issues that need to be addressed as part of medical training. Practitioners need to be aware of the implications relating to professional liability, informed patient consent, and the regulatory standards governing this innovative practice.
e. **Impact on access to care:** Finally, a fundamental aspect of telesurgery's impact is its potential to improve access to medical care in remote or underserved areas. Training must therefore also address how to use these technologies to optimize clinical outcomes, while taking into account geographical disparities in access to care.

III. Clinical applications and benefits of robotics

Robot-assisted surgery is a major advance in the medical field, offering innovative solutions for a variety of surgical procedures. This technology uses robotic systems to help surgeons perform operations with increased precision, reduced tissue trauma and faster recovery times for patients. In-depth studies on this technology highlight its varied clinical applications, its benefits, as well as the challenges associated with its use.

Clinical applications of robot-assisted surgery

- **Urological surgery**: Robot-assisted prostatectomy is one of the most common applications. Studies show that this method reduces blood loss and improves post-operative functional recovery (Menon et al., 2007).

- **Gynecological surgery**: procedures such as hysterectomies can be performed with greater precision thanks to robotics, enabling surgeons to access difficult areas while minimizing incisions (Miller et al., 2010).

- **Thoracic surgery**: the use of robots in thoracic procedures has improved visualization and access to lung structures, resulting in fewer post-operative complications (D'Ancona et al., 2014).

- **Orthopedic surgery**: robotic systems are used to guide surgeons during joint replacements, ensuring precise alignment of implants (Baker et al., 2016).

- **Pediatric surgery**: robot-assisted surgery is also used in children, where it enables complex procedures to be performed with less physical stress on the patient (Kumar et al., 2018).

Benefits of robotics in surgery: Advantages associated with the use of robot-assisted surgery include:

- **Improved precision**: robotic arms offer greater stability than human hands, enabling finer movements.

- **Less invasiveness**: Minimally invasive techniques reduce tissue trauma, resulting in less post-operative pain and shorter hospital stays.

- **Rapid recovery**: Patients undergoing robot-assisted surgery generally show a faster return to normal activities.

- **Enhanced visualization**: The technology enables better three-dimensional visualization of the surgical field, helping the surgeon to make informed decisions during the operation.

- **Advanced training for surgeons**: Robotic systems also offer platforms for continuing education for medical professionals, enabling them to improve their surgical skills.

Challenges associated with robot-assisted surgery: Despite its many advantages, there are several challenges associated with the widespread adoption of robot-assisted surgery:

- **High cost**: acquiring and maintaining robotic systems represents a significant investment for medical establishments.

- **Learning curve**: Mastering robotic systems requires specialized training, which can take time.

- **Technological limitations**: Although technology is advanced, it is not infallible; there is always a risk of technical failure during surgery.

Practical work: Robotic Assistance in the Surgical Management of Endometriosis

Introduction

Endometriosis is a chronic gynecological disease that affects a significant proportion of women of childbearing age. It is characterized by the presence of endometrial tissue outside the uterus, leading to pain, infertility and other complications. The surgical management of endometriosis has evolved thanks to the integration of robotic technologies, offering significant advantages over traditional surgical techniques.

Practical work objectives

- **Understanding the Basics of Endometriosis**: Students will research the causes, symptoms and clinical implications of endometriosis.
- **Exploring Traditional Surgical Techniques**: An analysis of conventional methods used to treat endometriosis, including laparoscopy.
- **Analyze the Role of Robotics**: Study how robotic systems, such as the Da Vinci Surgical System, improve surgical precision and reduce recovery time.
- **Assess Advantages and Disadvantages**: Discuss benefits (such as better visualization and less postoperative pain) as well as potential limitations (high costs, learning curve).

- **Case studies**: Analyze recent studies demonstrating the effectiveness of robotic interventions in the treatment of endometriosis.

Methodology

Students will be expected to carry out extensive bibliographical research on the above-mentioned topics. They should use academic articles, specialized books and medical journals to support their analyses.

Conclusion

This practical work aims to raise students' awareness of the growing importance of robotic technology in the medical field, particularly in gynecological surgery. Through this exploration, they will develop a critical understanding of technological innovations and their impact on women's health.

Chapter 7: Minimally invasive surgery

Introduction

Minimally invasive surgery, also known as laparoscopic or endoscopic surgery, is a surgical approach that uses less invasive techniques than traditional surgery. This method has gained in popularity over the last few decades thanks to its many advantages for both patients and surgeons. The main aim of minimally invasive surgery is to reduce tissue trauma, speed up post-operative recovery and improve overall patient outcomes.

History and development

Minimally invasive surgery began to emerge in the 1980s with the introduction of laparoscopy. This type of surgery uses specialized instruments and a camera inserted through small incisions in the body, enabling surgeons to visualize and operate on internal organs without the need for a large incision. Over time, this technique has been adapted for a variety of surgical procedures, including cholecystectomy (removal of the gallbladder), hysterectomy (removal of the uterus) and even some cardiac interventions.

Advantages of minimally invasive surgery: The advantages associated with minimally invasive surgery are manifold:

- **Less pain**: Smaller incisions generally entail less post-operative pain than larger incisions.
- **Faster recovery**: Patients can often leave hospital sooner and resume their daily activities more quickly.
- **Fewer complications**: The risk of infections and other complications is often reduced thanks to minimal tissue trauma.
- **Better aesthetics**: Scars resulting from small incisions are generally less visible.

Modern techniques

As technology has advanced, a number of techniques have been developed to further enhance minimally invasive surgery. Surgical robotics, for example, enable greater precision thanks to computer-controlled instruments that offer improved maneuverability and a three-dimensional view of the operating field. In addition, the use of tools such as advanced imaging devices helps surgeons to plan and execute complex procedures with greater efficiency.

Conclusion

Minimally invasive surgery represents a significant change in the medical field, offering patients safer and less painful options for treating a variety of medical conditions. As this discipline continues to evolve with technological innovation, it is essential for healthcare professionals to keep abreast of these developments in order to offer the best possible care.

I. Endoscopic and laparoscopic techniques

Endoscopic techniques represent a significant advance in modern medicine, enabling doctors to explore the inside of the human body without the need for invasive surgery. Endoscopy uses an instrument called an endoscope, which is a flexible tube equipped with a camera and lights, enabling direct visualization of internal organs. This method is widely used to diagnose and treat a variety of medical conditions, notably in the fields of gastroenterology, pneumology and urology.

1. History and development of endoscopic techniques

The history of endoscopy goes back several centuries, but it wasn't until the 20th century that techniques were truly developed thanks to technological advances. The first endoscopes were rigid and limited in use. With the introduction of fiber optics in the 1950s, it became possible to create more flexible instruments that could navigate the human body with greater ease.

2. **Types of endoscopy:** There are several types of endoscopy, each tailored to specific parts of the body:

- **Gastroscopy**: to examine the oesophagus, stomach and duodenum.
- **Colonoscopy**: to inspect the colon and rectum.
- **Bronchoscopy**: to visualize the respiratory tract.
- **Cystoscopy**: to examine the bladder.

Each type of endoscopy has its own clinical indications, contraindications and specific protocols.

3. **Endoscopic procedure**

The procedure usually begins with adequate patient preparation, which may include fasting or bowel preparation depending on the type of examination. During the examination, the patient may receive mild sedation to minimize discomfort. The endoscope is then inserted via the natural route (mouth or anus) or through a small incision if necessary.

4. **Therapeutic applications**

In addition to diagnosis, endoscopic techniques also allow therapeutic interventions such as :

- Biopsy (tissue sampling).
- Electrocoagulation (to stop bleeding).
- Dilatation of stenoses (narrowings).

These procedures often minimize the need for open surgery and considerably reduce recovery time.

5. **Recent advances**

Recent research is focusing on improving imaging technologies used in endoscopy, including the use of robotic systems and artificial intelligence to improve diagnostic accuracy and reduce the risks associated with procedures.

A. Endoscopy

Endoscopy is a medical technique that uses an instrument called an endoscope to explore the inside of the human body. This method is used to diagnose and treat a variety of medical conditions, notably in the fields of gastroenterology, pneumology, ear, nose and throat (ENT), and surgery. In-depth, hands-on study of modern endoscopy techniques encompasses many aspects, including technological advances, clinical applications, safety protocols, and training for healthcare professionals.

1. The history of the development of endoscopic techniques

Endoscopy is a medical technique used to explore the inside of the human body using an instrument called an endoscope. The history of the development of endoscopic techniques goes back several centuries, with significant contributions coming from various fields such as medicine, physics and engineering.

Historical origins: The earliest forms of endoscopy can be traced back to antiquity. Greek physicians used rudimentary instruments to examine body cavities. However, it was in the 19th century that the modern foundations of endoscopy were laid. In 1806, German physician Philipp Bozzini developed a device called the "Lichtleiter" (light conductor), which enabled body cavities to be explored using light. This device was limited by the technology of the time, but it paved the way for future innovations.

Technological developments: Over the course of the 20th century, a number of technological advances have revolutionized the field of endoscopy. The introduction of fiber optics in the 1950s gave doctors better visualization of internal organs. Fiber optics enabled light and images to be transmitted from inside the body to an external screen, considerably improving the quality of examinations.

At the same time, the development of video cameras and digital imaging systems has also played a crucial role in the evolution of endoscopy. These technologies have enabled not only better real-time visualization, but also more efficient recording and documentation of medical procedures.

Clinical applications: Endoscopic techniques have become essential in a variety of medical fields, including gastroenterology, pulmonology and urology. For example, gastroscopy is used to examine the oesophagus, stomach and duodenum to diagnose conditions such as ulcers or cancer. Similarly, colonoscopy is used to examine the colon for polyps and other abnormalities.

Interventional endoscopy has also emerged as a specialty in its own right, enabling not only diagnosis but also treatment of certain conditions without the need for invasive surgery. Procedures such as endoluminal dilatation or stenting are now commonplace.

Future prospects

With continuing advances in medical and computer technologies, we can expect endoscopic techniques to continue to evolve. The integration of artificial intelligence to aid diagnosis and image analysis could further transform this discipline.

2. Advanced studies in endoscopy

Endoscopy studies include both theoretical and practical training. Training programs vary from country to country, but generally include courses on human anatomy, physiology and pathology, as well as specific modules on endoscopic techniques. Students also learn how to interpret the results of endoscopic examinations and manage potential complications.

- **Theoretical training**: This includes courses on the fundamentals of endoscopy, including an understanding of the different types of endoscopes (rigid and flexible), how they work, and the indications and contraindications of endoscopic procedures.

- **Hands-on training**: Students must gain practical experience under supervision. This may include simulations on models or mannequins before moving on to actual procedures on patients. Hands-on experience is crucial to developing the manual dexterity needed for precise endoscope use.

- **Skills required**: Key skills include not only technical handling of the endoscope, but also communication with the patient, stress management in clinical situations, and the ability to work effectively as part of a multidisciplinary medical team.

- **Continuous assessment**: Professionals often have to go through a process of continuous assessment to keep their skills up to date. This can include additional training, hands-on workshops, and even specific certifications based on technological advances in the field.

- **Research and development**: Endoscopy is a constantly evolving field, with new technologies and techniques being introduced on a regular basis. Consequently, it is essential that practitioners engage in ongoing research to keep abreast of best practice.

Skills required: Skills required to practice endoscopy include:

- **Technical skills**: Ability to handle various endoscopic instruments.
- **Analytical skills**: Precise interpretation of images obtained during examinations.
- **Interpersonal skills**: Effective communication with patients before, during and after procedures.
- **Time management**: Ability to carry out procedures within a given timeframe while maintaining a high level of quality.
- **Problem solving**: Ability to anticipate and manage complications that may arise during a procedure.

3. Risks and Complications in Endoscopy

✓ **Mechanical complications**: Mechanical complications include perforation of internal organs, which can occur during insertion of the endoscope or during manipulation of the endoscope. Perforation can lead to leakage of intestinal contents into the abdominal cavity, resulting in peritonitis.

- ✓ **Bleeding**: Bleeding is another potential complication, especially during procedures such as polypectomy or biopsy. Bleeding may be minor or require surgery to control.

- ✓ **Infections**: Infections can occur after endoscopy due to bacterial contamination during the procedure. This is of particular concern in the case of gastrointestinal endoscopy, where intestinal bacteria can enter the bloodstream.

- ✓ **Reactions to anesthetics**: The use of sedative or general anesthetics also presents risks. Allergic reactions or respiratory complications may occur in some patients.

- ✓ **Endoscopy-specific risks**: Each type of endoscopy has its own specific risks. For example, bronchial endoscopy can lead to bronchial spasm or hypoxia, while urological endoscopy can cause kidney damage.

Risk management: To minimize these risks, it is essential that physicians carry out a thorough pre-operative assessment of the patient, including a detailed physical examination and complete medical history. In addition, informed consent must be obtained after discussing potential benefits and risks with the patient.

Rigorous sterilization protocols for endoscopic equipment are also crucial in preventing post-procedural infections. Finally, appropriate post-operative monitoring ensures early detection of any complications.

4. Future innovations in endoscopy

Endoscopy is a medical technique used to explore the inside of the human body using an instrument called an endoscope. This method has evolved significantly over recent decades, thanks to technological advances and innovations in the medical field. In-depth studies on future innovations in endoscopy focus on several areas, including instrument improvements, the integration of new technologies, and the optimization of clinical procedures.

- o **Technological innovations:** Recent innovations in endoscopy include the development of more flexible and miniaturized endoscopes, enabling access to previously inaccessible areas. For example, capsule endoscopes have become popular for their ability to capture images of the small intestine without the need for anesthesia or sedation. In addition, augmented reality (AR) and virtual reality (VR) technology is beginning to be integrated into endoscopic procedures to enhance visualization and navigation.

- **Artificial Intelligence (AI):** Artificial intelligence is playing a growing role in modern endoscopy. Machine learning algorithms are used to analyze endoscopic images to detect abnormalities such as polyps or early cancers with greater accuracy. These systems can help doctors make more informed decisions during procedures.
- **Minimally invasive techniques:** Endoscopy techniques are evolving towards less invasive approaches that reduce recovery time and minimize pain for the patient. Procedures such as interventional endoscopy allow not only diagnosis but also immediate treatment of certain conditions, such as dilatation of strictures or early detection of tumors.
- **Training and education:** Ongoing training of healthcare professionals is essential to integrate these new technologies into clinical practice. Educational programs using simulation and AR are being developed to effectively train doctors in new endoscopic techniques.
- **Future prospects:** Future prospects for innovation in endoscopy include the increased use of nanotechnologies to develop even smaller tools capable of performing diagnostics at the cellular level, as well as the continued improvement of fluorescence and contrast imaging for better intra-operative visualization.

B. Laparoscopy

1. The history and development of laparoscopic techniques

Laparoscopy, a minimally invasive surgical technique, has undergone significant development since its inception. Its history dates back to the early 20th century, when the first abdominal explorations were performed using rigid tubes and light. However, it was in the 1980s that laparoscopy really took off, with the introduction of laparoscopic cholecystectomy, which revolutionized the treatment of gallbladder disease.

History and development

- **Origins**: The first attempts at laparoscopic surgery can be traced back to 1910, when Austrian surgeon Georg Kelling performed the first laparoscopic abdominal exploration. He used an instrument called a "trocar" to insert a tube into the abdominal cavity.

- **Technological advances**: In the 1930s, the development of more sophisticated instruments and improved light sources enabled surgeons to explore the abdomen more effectively. However, these techniques were not widely adopted due to technological limitations.

- **Revolution of the 1980s**: The real revolution came with laparoscopic cholecystectomy performed by Dr. Philippe Mouret in France in 1987. This procedure demonstrated the advantages of laparoscopic surgery, including faster recovery and fewer post-operative complications.

- **Expanding indications**: Over the years, the indications for laparoscopic surgery have broadened to include not only abdominal procedures, but also thoracic and gynecological procedures. Techniques such as robot-assisted laparoscopy have also emerged, further enhancing the precision and efficiency of operations.

- **Training and Practice**: Training in laparoscopic techniques has become essential for modern surgeons. Specialized programs have been set up to teach these skills to future practitioners to ensure safe and effective adoption of these surgical methods.

- **Impact on surgical practice**: The rise of laparoscopic surgery has had a profound impact on contemporary surgical practice, altering not only operative approaches but also patients' expectations of their recovery from surgery.

2. Laparascopic techniques

Laparoscopic techniques involve the use of a laparoscope, a camera-equipped instrument that enables surgeons to view the inside of the body on a screen. Common procedures include cholecystectomy (removal of the gallbladder), appendectomy (removal of the appendix) and various gynecological operations. Training in laparoscopic techniques involves not only theoretical learning but also extensive hands-on practice on simulators and anatomical models.

Laparoscopic instruments: The instruments used in laparoscopy are specific and include:

- **Laparoscope**: A thin tube with a camera at the end.
- **Trocar**: An instrument used to create an opening in the abdominal wall.

- **Laparoscopic forceps and scissors**: Used to manipulate tissue.
- **Endoscopic sutures**: To close internal incisions.
- **Energy devices**: Like electrobistouris, which cut and coagulate tissue.

Training and Practice: Training in laparoscopic techniques is crucial to ensure patient safety and successful operations. Surgeons must go through rigorous training programs that include:

- **Theoretical training**: Courses on anatomy, physiology and surgical principles.
- **Simulation**: Use of simulators to practice skills without risk to patients.
- **Mentoring**: Observation and assistance during actual procedures under the supervision of an experienced surgeon.

Laparoscopic instruments: The instruments used in laparoscopy are specific and include:

- **Laparoscope**: A thin tube with a camera at the end.
- **Trocar**: An instrument used to create an opening in the abdominal wall.
- **Laparoscopic forceps and scissors**: Used to manipulate tissue.
- **Endoscopic sutures**: To close internal incisions.
- **Energy devices**: Like electrobistouris, which cut and coagulate tissue.

3. The advantages and disadvantages of laparoscopy

Advantages of laparoscopy

- **Less post-operative pain**: Patients undergoing laparoscopic surgery generally experience less pain after the procedure than those who have undergone open surgery. This is due to the reduced size of the incisions, resulting in less trauma to the surrounding tissue.

- **Faster recovery**: Recovery from laparoscopic surgery is often faster. Patients can usually return to their daily activities in a shorter time, reducing hospitalization time and associated costs.

- **Fewer complications**: Studies show that laparoscopy can lead to fewer post-operative complications, such as infections and bleeding, compared with open surgery.

- **Better visualization**: The laparoscope gives surgeons an enlarged, illuminated view of the inside of the body, which can improve the precision of surgical interventions.

- **Improved aesthetics**: the smaller incisions used in laparoscopy often result in less visible scarring, which can be an important factor for some patients.

Disadvantages of laparoscopy

- **Technical limitations**: Although laparoscopy is effective for many procedures, some complex interventions may not be feasible using this method due to technical or anatomical limitations.

- **Specific risks**: As with any surgical procedure, laparoscopy entails specific risks, such as injury to internal organs or blood vessels during instrument insertion.

- **High costs**: The initial cost of the equipment needed to perform laparoscopic surgery can be high, which can be a problem in some healthcare systems or medical establishments.

- **Learning curve**: Mastering laparoscopic techniques requires specialized training and significant experience; surgeons must develop their skills to minimize the risks associated with this approach.

- **Potential failure**: In some cases, if complications arise during the operation or if the surgeon encounters technical difficulties, it may be necessary to convert the procedure to open surgery, thereby negating some of the initial advantages.

4. Clinical applications

The clinical applications of laparoscopy are varied. They include :

- **Gynecological surgery**: Laparoscopy is commonly used to treat conditions such as endometriosis, uterine fibroids and to perform hysterectomies.
- **Digestive surgery**: used to perform cholecystectomies (removal of the gallbladder), appendectomies and even more complex procedures such as bariatric surgery.
- **Urological surgery**: Procedures such as nephrectomy (removal of the kidney) can be performed laparoscopically.

5. Training and skills required for laparoscopy

Required training

- **Basic Medical Education**: Surgeons must first obtain a medical degree (MD or DO) followed by residency training in their chosen specialty. This usually includes training in general surgery before further specialization.

- **Specialized Laparoscopic Training**: After completing their residency, physicians can pursue fellowship programs specifically focused on laparoscopic surgery. These programs offer advanced training in laparoscopic techniques, management of complications and use of associated technologies.

- **Continuing education**: As surgical techniques evolve rapidly with technological advances, it is crucial that practitioners attend continuing education courses, workshops and conferences to keep up to date with new methods and technologies.

Skills required

- **Technical skills**: Surgeons need to master several technical skills specific to laparoscopy, such as precise manipulation of instruments through small incisions, control of the camera during the operation, and the execution of internal sutures.

- **Problem-solving skills**: The ability to anticipate and manage complications that may arise during laparoscopic surgery is crucial. This requires a solid anatomical understanding as well as practical experience.

- **Interpersonal skills**: Surgeons also need excellent interpersonal skills to communicate effectively with their medical teams as well as with their patients before and after procedures.

- **Technological adaptability**: With the increasing integration of new technologies such as augmented reality and robotic systems into the surgical field, it is essential that practitioners are able to learn these new tools quickly.

- **Critical appraisal of data**: Professionals must be able to evaluate evidence-based clinical outcomes in order to continually improve their surgical practices.

Practical work: Endoscopic surgery for herniated lobar discs

Endoscopic lumbar disc herniation surgery is a minimally invasive surgical technique that treats herniated discs using an endoscope. This method offers several advantages over traditional open surgery, including reduced postoperative pain, shorter recovery time and fewer complications. As part of a practical assignment for students, it is essential to explore the technical, clinical and theoretical aspects of this procedure.

Objectives :

- Understand the anatomy and pathophysiology of herniated lumbar discs.
- Study the indications and contraindications of endoscopic surgery.
- Analyze surgical techniques used in endoscopic surgery.
- Evaluate clinical outcomes and potential complications associated with this procedure.

Work structure :

- **Introduction**
  - Definition of herniated lumbar discs.
  - Importance of endoscopic surgery in treatment.

- **Anatomy and Pathophysiology**
    - Description of the intervertebral discs and their role.
    - Mechanisms of disc herniation.
- **Indications and contraindications**
    - Criteria for choosing endoscopic surgery over other treatments.
    - Situations where surgery is not recommended.
- **Surgical techniques**
    - Details of equipment used (endoscope, specific instruments).
    - Steps in the surgical procedure (access, decompression, closure).
- **Clinical results**
    - Analysis of recent studies on the effectiveness of endoscopic surgery.
    - Comparison with other surgical methods (open surgery).
- **Potential Complications**
    - Discussion of the risks associated with endoscopic surgery.
    - Strategies to minimize these risks.

Conclusion

Summary of the advantages and disadvantages of the technique.

Future prospects for this surgical approach.

II. Advantages and disadvantages of minimally invasive approaches

Minimally invasive approaches, encompassing a variety of surgical and medical techniques, have gained in popularity over the past few decades. These methods are distinguished by their ability to reduce tissue trauma, minimize postoperative pain and promote faster recovery compared to traditional surgical procedures. However, it is essential to examine the advantages and disadvantages associated with these techniques to assess their effectiveness in a variety of clinical settings.

Advantages of Mini-Invasive Approaches

- **Reduced Tissue Trauma**: Minimally invasive procedures often use small incisions or endoscopic techniques, resulting in less damage to surrounding tissue. This can shorten healing time and reduce the risk of post-operative infections.

- **Less post-operative pain**: Patients undergoing minimally invasive procedures generally report less post-operative pain. This can be attributed to reduced tissue trauma, as well as the use of regional or local rather than general anesthetics.

- **Rapid recovery**: Thanks to the less invasive nature of these procedures, patients can often return to their daily activities more quickly than those who have undergone traditional surgery. This has positive implications not only for the patient's quality of life, but also for overall healthcare costs.

- **Less scarring**: The small incisions used in minimally invasive techniques generally result in less visible scarring, which is an important factor for many patients.

- **Reduced hospitalization**: Many minimally invasive procedures can be performed on an outpatient basis, reducing the need for prolonged hospitalization and lowering the costs associated with hospital care.

Disadvantages of Mini-Invasive Approaches

- **Technical limitations**: Certain medical or anatomical conditions may make it difficult to apply minimally invasive techniques. For example, in some complex cases, a traditional approach may be required to ensure an optimal result.

- **Surgical skill required**: Mastering minimally invasive techniques requires specialized training and significant experience. Not all surgeons possess these skills, which may limit access to these methods for some patients.

- **High costs**: Although overall costs may be reduced thanks to faster recovery, the initial cost of the equipment needed to perform these procedures can be high, which could pose a problem in some medical institutions.

- **Specific associated risks**: Like any medical intervention, minimally invasive approaches carry their own specific risks, such as the possibility of conversion to open surgery if complications arise during the procedure.

- **Limited Long-Term Evaluation**: Although many studies show positive short-term results with mini- invasive approaches, there is still a need for longitudinal evaluations to fully understand their long-term health effects.

III. clinical practice and modern equipment

1. Historical development and theoretical foundations

The first minimally invasive surgery techniques date back to the 1980s, with the introduction of laparoscopy. Surgeons began using specialized instruments to perform surgery through small incisions, revolutionizing the surgical field. Extensive studies on the physiological and psychological effects of this approach have shown that patients benefit from shorter hospital stays and a quicker return to daily activities.

2. Techniques and procedures

Common procedures in minimally invasive surgery include laparoscopic cholecystectomy (gallbladder removal), laparoscopic appendectomy (appendix removal) and various gynecological interventions. These techniques require specialized training for surgeons to ensure their proficiency in using delicate instruments and navigating the human anatomy with precision.

3. Modern equipment

The equipment used in minimally invasive surgery has evolved considerably. Advanced imaging systems, such as high-definition cameras and real-time imaging devices, enable surgeons to visualize the surgical site with exceptional clarity. In addition, surgical robots, such as the da Vinci system, offer enhanced precision thanks to robotic arms that mimic human movements while reducing tremor.

4. Evidence-based clinical practice

Recent research has focused on the effectiveness of minimally invasive techniques compared with traditional methods. Randomized clinical trials have demonstrated that these approaches result in fewer post-operative complications and a better return to quality of life for patients. Statistical analysis of results enables clinicians to adapt their practices based on evidence.

5. Future prospects

The future of minimally invasive surgery looks bright, with the continued integration of new technologies such as augmented reality and artificial intelligence to further enhance surgical precision. Ongoing research in this field aims to refine these techniques to broaden their application to a wider range of surgical procedures.

Practical work: Laparoscopic uretero-vesical anastomosis stimulation on a training model

Laparoscopic uretero-vesical anastomosis stimulation on a training model is an advanced surgical technique that requires a thorough understanding of anatomical principles, surgical techniques and postoperative considerations. This type of hands-on work is essential for medical and surgical students to develop their practical skills and confidence in a controlled environment before moving on to actual clinical procedures.

Practical work objectives

- **Anatomical Understanding**: Students must first acquire a sound knowledge of the anatomy of the urinary system, including the location of the ureters, bladder and surrounding structures. This includes identification of relevant blood vessels, nerves and connective tissues.

- **Laparoscopic techniques**: Students should become familiar with the laparoscopic instruments used to perform a uretero-vesical anastomosis. This includes handling the camera, using forceps, scissors and other tools specific to laparoscopy.

- **Practical simulation**: Use a training model (often made of silicone or synthetic fabric) that reproduces human anatomical features to enable students to practice anastomosis without risk to a real patient . This model should be designed to simulate the challenges encountered during actual surgery.

- **Surgical procedure**: Key steps in uretero-vesical anastomosis include:

  - Delicate dissection of the ureters.
  - Preparation of the edges of the ureters and bladder.
  - The use of absorbable or non-absorbable sutures to perform the anastomosis.
  - Verification of anastomosis tightness by saline injection or other appropriate method.

- **Post-operative evaluation**: After performing the anastomosis, it's crucial that students learn to evaluate the success of their procedure through simulated clinical examinations, including the detection of possible complications such as urinary leakage or infection.

Methodolog

- **Theoretical sessions**: Prior to practical work, it is recommended that students attend theoretical sessions on laparoscopic surgery and the anatomical specifics of uretero-vesical anastomosis.

- **Practical Workshops**: Organize several workshops where students can practice under direct supervision. Each student should have access to his or her own training model to maximize hands-on time.

- **Constructive feedback**: After each practical session, provide detailed feedback on individual performance so that each student can identify his or her strengths and areas for improvement.

Evaluation

Assessment can take the form of a practical examination in which each student must demonstrate his or her ability to perform a uretero-vesical anastomosis on the training model, while adhering to the appropriate surgical protocols.

Chapter 8: Image-guided surgery

Introduction

Image-guided surgery is a medical discipline that uses imaging techniques to improve the precision and efficiency of surgical interventions. This approach enables surgeons to visualize anatomical structures in real time, which is essential for minimizing damage to surrounding tissue and optimizing clinical outcomes. The use of imaging technologies such as ultrasound, computed tomography (CT), magnetic resonance imaging (MRI) and fluoroscopy has revolutionized the surgical field, offering precise information on lesion location, vascularization and other critical anatomical features.

One of the main advantages of image-guided surgery is its ability to reduce the risk of post-operative complications. By providing direct visualization of internal structures, this technique enables surgeons to plan their interventions with greater precision. For example, in the case of solid tumors, images can help determine appropriate excision margins, ensuring that the entire tumor is removed while preserving as much healthy tissue as possible.

Image-guided surgery also favours the development of less invasive procedures. Endoscopic and laparoscopic techniques benefit greatly from advances in imaging, enabling surgeons to perform operations with smaller incisions and reduced recovery time for patients. This represents a significant advance in the surgical field, improving not only clinical outcomes but also the overall patient experience.

Another important aspect of this discipline is its growing integration with other advanced technologies such as robotics and artificial intelligence. These innovations enable better handling of surgical instruments under precise visual guidance, increasing the safety and efficiency of procedures.

In short, image-guided surgery represents a major advance in the medical field. It combines advanced technology and surgical expertise to deliver improved patient care. As these technologies continue to evolve, it is likely that their impact on surgical practice will become even more significant.

I. Use of real-time imaging (MRI, CT Scan)

Real-time imaging, notably through the use of Magnetic Resonance Imaging (MRI) and Computed Tomography (CT scan), has revolutionized the medical field by offering non-invasive methods for visualizing the internal structures of the human body. These techniques enable doctors to diagnose and treat a variety of conditions with greater precision.

1. Magnetic Resonance Imaging (MRI)

Magnetic Resonance Imaging (MRI) is a medical imaging technique that uses powerful magnetic fields and radio waves to produce detailed images of organs and tissues inside the body. This method is non-invasive and does not require the use of ionizing radiation, making it a preferred choice for medical diagnosis.

In-depth MRI studies

- **Physical principles**: MRI is based on the principle of nuclear magnetic resonance (NMR). Atomic nuclei, particularly the hydrogen nuclei found in the water molecules of the human body, are excited by an external magnetic field. When this field is applied, the nuclei absorb energy and move to a higher energy state. When they return to their ground state, they emit a signal that can be detected and transformed into an image.

- **Imaging sequences**: The different MRI sequences (such as T1, T2, FLAIR) enable us to highlight different types of tissue and pathologies. For example, the T1 sequence is often used to visualize normal anatomy, while the T2 sequence is more sensitive to pathological changes such as edema or lesions.

- **Clinical applications**: MRI is widely used in various medical specialties such as neurology (to detect brain tumors or strokes), orthopedics (to examine joints and soft tissues), and cardiology (to assess cardiac structure).

- **Technological advances**: Recent advances in MRI include functional MRI (fMRI), which measures changes in blood flow related to neuronal activity, and diffusion imaging techniques that assess tissue microstructure.

- **Challenges and limitations**: Despite its many advantages, MRI has certain limitations, such as the high cost of equipment, the length of examinations, and certain contraindications, such as the presence of metal implants in certain patients.

MRI practices: Clinical practices around MRI involve not only the technical operation of the device, but also a thorough understanding of the appropriate clinical indications for its use. Ongoing training of radiologists and imaging technicians is essential to ensure accurate interpretation of results.

Advantages of MRI :

- **High resolution**: MRI offers superior spatial resolution for highly detailed images.
- **Tissue contrast**: It provides excellent contrast between different types of tissue, which is essential for identifying abnormalities.
- **Functional imaging**: advanced techniques such as functional MRI (fMRI) can assess brain activity by measuring changes in blood flow.

Limitations:

- **High cost**: MRI equipment is expensive to acquire and maintain.
- **Examination time**: Examinations may take longer than other imaging modalities.
- **Contraindications**: Patients with certain metal implants or claustrophobias may not be eligible for this procedure.

2. Computed tomography (CT scan)

Computed tomography (CT) is a medical imaging technique that uses X-rays to create detailed images of the body's internal structures. This method is widely used in medical diagnostics due to its ability to provide cross-sectional images, enabling precise visualization of organs, tissues and blood vessels.

Principles of computed tomography

The fundamental principle of CT scanning is based on the use of an X-ray tube that rotates around the patient. As the tube emits X-rays, a detector opposite captures the rays as they pass through the body. The data collected is then processed by a computer to generate cross-sectional images. These images can be reconstructed from different angles and viewed in 2D or 3D.

Clinical applications: The clinical applications of CT are vast and include:

- **Tumor diagnosis**: CT scanning is essential for detecting and characterizing tumors in various organs such as the lungs, liver and pancreas.

- **Traumatological assessment**: In the event of trauma, particularly cranial or abdominal, CT scanning can quickly identify internal bleeding or bone fractures.

- **Surgical planning**: Before certain surgical procedures, a CT scan can help plan the surgical approach by providing a detailed view of the local anatomy.

- **Therapeutic follow-up**: It is also used to monitor the evolution of diseases such as cancer after treatment, in order to evaluate the effectiveness of the treatment.

- **Vascular imaging**: Angiographic CT scans examine blood vessels and can help diagnose conditions such as aneurysms or thrombosis.

Advantages of CT scanning :

- **Speed**: CT examinations are generally fast, which is crucial in emergency situations.
- **Bone visualization**: CT scanning is particularly effective for visualizing bone fractures and internal lesions.
- **Multi-system evaluation**: Allows rapid, comprehensive evaluation of multiple body systems.

Limitations:

- **Radiation exposure** : The CT scan exposes the patient to a significant dose of ionizing radiation, which may pose an increased risk if used frequently.
- **Less tissue contrast than MRI**: While effective for certain structures, it may not offer the same level of detail as MRI for soft tissues.

II. Surgical navigation techniques

Surgical navigation is a technology that enables surgeons to visualize the patient's anatomy in real time, improving the precision of interventions and reducing the risks associated with surgery. This approach uses positioning and imaging systems to guide surgical instruments with great accuracy.

1. The history and development of surgical navigation techniques

Surgical navigation is an evolving discipline that combines modern technology with the fundamental principles of surgery. Its history dates back several decades, but it has experienced significant growth thanks to recent technological advances. Surgical navigation uses imaging and localization systems to guide surgeons during operations, improving precision and reducing the risks associated with surgery.

Origins and evolution: The first forms of surgical navigation were developed in the 1980s with the introduction of magnetic resonance imaging (MRI) and computed tomography (CT) systems. These technologies enabled surgeons to obtain precise images of the internal structures of the human body before performing an operation. As these technologies have been perfected, they have been integrated into navigation systems that enable real-time visualization during surgery.

Technologies used : Modern surgical navigation techniques are based on several key technologies:

- **Medical imaging**: MRI, CT and ultrasound are commonly used to create three-dimensional models of anatomical structures.
- **Localization systems**: Optical or electromagnetic sensors are used to track the position of surgical instruments in real time.
- **Advanced software**: Sophisticated algorithms enable rapid processing of imaging data, providing surgeons with a precise, dynamic view of the surgical site.

Clinical Applications: Surgical navigation is used in a variety of medical specialties, including :

- **Neurosurgery**: to pinpoint the precise location of brain tumors or vascular anomalies.
- **Orthopedics**: for joint implants where millimetric precision is crucial.

- **Oncological surgery**: To effectively remove tumors while preserving the surrounding healthy tissue.

Benefits and challenges : The benefits of surgical navigation include:

- ✓ **Improved accuracy**: Reduced human error thanks to precise visual guidance.
- ✓ **Fewer complications**: Reduced risk of damage to surrounding tissue.
- ✓ **Accelerated recovery**: Patients can benefit from less invasive procedures.
- ✓ However, there are also challenges:
- ✓ **High cost**: Navigation systems can be expensive to acquire and maintain.
- ✓ **Training required**: Surgeons need to be trained to use these technologies effectively.

2. Technologies used in surgical navigation techniques

These technologies enable surgeons to visualize and navigate precisely through the patient's anatomy, which is particularly crucial in complex procedures such as neurosurgery, orthopedic surgery and other specialties.

1. Introduction to surgical navigation

Surgical navigation uses positioning and imaging systems to guide surgical instruments with increased precision. Navigation systems can integrate various imaging modalities, including MRI (magnetic resonance imaging), CT (computed tomography), and ultrasound, enabling three-dimensional representation of anatomical structures.

2. Key technologies : Key technologies used in surgical navigation techniques include:

- **Localization systems**: These systems use optical or electromagnetic sensors to track surgical instruments in real time.
- **Pre-operative imaging**: The use of pre-operative images enables surgeons to plan their interventions with a better understanding of anatomical structures.

- **3D modeling**: The creation of three-dimensional models from medical images helps to simulate the procedure before it is performed on the patient.

3. Clinical applications: The clinical applications of surgical navigation techniques are vast:

- **Neurosurgery**: In brain surgery, navigation enables neurosurgeons to access critical areas while minimizing damage to healthy tissue.
- **Orthopaedic surgery**: procedures such as joint replacements benefit greatly from the precision offered by these technologies.
- **Oncology surgery**: Navigation helps to locate and precisely remove tumors while preserving surrounding healthy tissue.

4. Benefits and challenges

Benefits include reduced operating time, lower risk of complications, and improved post-operative functional results. However, there are also challenges such as the high cost of equipment, the need for specialized training for medical staff, and potential problems related to technological integration in operating rooms.

3. The advantages and challenges of surgical navigation techniques

Advantages of Surgical Navigation Techniques

- **Improved precision**: One of the key benefits of surgical navigation techniques is the significant increase in precision during surgery. Navigation systems enable surgeons to pinpoint the exact location of critical anatomical structures, minimizing the risk of damaging surrounding tissue. In orthopedic surgery, for example, computer-aided navigation enables more precise placement of implants.

- **Pre-operative planning**: The ability to create 3D models based on pre-operative imagery enables surgeons to plan their operations in great detail. This includes evaluating the best surgical approaches and simulating complex procedures before they are carried out.

- **Reduced operating time**: By providing real-time guidance, these systems can reduce the time needed to perform certain surgical procedures. This can also reduce anesthesia time and stress on the patient.

- **Improved Clinical Outcomes**: Studies have shown that the use of surgical navigation techniques can lead to a lower rate of post-operative complications, such as infections or errors in implant placement.

- **Training and education**: Navigation systems also provide a platform for the continuing education of surgeons, enabling them to improve their skills in a controlled environment before applying these techniques on real patients.

Challenges of Surgical Navigation Techniques

- **High costs**: One of the main drawbacks is the cost associated with acquiring and maintaining the equipment required for surgical navigation. These costs can be prohibitive for some medical establishments, limiting access to this advanced technology.

- **Learning curve**: Although these technologies are designed to improve surgical practice, they require specialized training to be used effectively. Surgeons must go through a learning curve that can vary according to their previous experience with digital technologies.

- **Technological dependence**: Another concern is the increasing dependence on technology during surgery. In the event of technical failure or system error, patient safety could be compromised.

- **Clinical integration**: Efficiently integrating navigation systems into the existing operational workflow can pose a significant logistical challenge for some hospitals or clinics, often requiring significant reorganization of staff and procedures.

- **Inter-operator variability**: The performance and efficiency of systems can vary considerably depending on the operator, raising questions about uniformity and standardization in their use within the same institution or between different institutions.

III. Application in orthopedic neurosurgery

Orthopedic neurosurgery is a specialized field that combines the principles of neurosurgery with those of orthopedics to treat conditions related to the spine, peripheral nerves and musculoskeletal structures. This discipline requires a thorough understanding of the central and peripheral nervous systems, as well as advanced surgical techniques.

1. Historical background and development

The evolution of orthopedic neurosurgery has been marked by significant technological advances, notably the introduction of advanced imaging tools such as MRI (magnetic resonance imaging) and CT scan (computed tomography). These technologies have enabled better visualization of anatomical structures, facilitating diagnosis and treatment of complex pathologies.

2. Surgical techniques

Surgical techniques in orthopedic neurosurgery include nerve decompression, spinal fusion and spinal tumor procedures. Nerve decompression is often performed to relieve pressure on nerves caused by herniated discs or spinal canal stenosis. Spinal fusion aims to stabilize the spine after surgery or injury.

3. Clinical applications

The clinical applications of orthopedic neurosurgery are vast. They encompass the treatment of conditions such as :

- Herniated discs
- Vertebral fractures
- Congenital malformations
- Spinal tumors
- Chronic pain syndromes

Each condition requires a personalized approach based on the patient's anatomy, the extent of the disease and post-operative functional goals.

4. Post-operative rehabilitation

Rehabilitation plays a crucial role in the success of orthopedic neurosurgical procedures. A well-structured rehabilitation program can help restore motor function, reduce pain and improve the patient's quality of life. This can include physical, occupational and psychological therapies.

5. Future prospects

With continued advances in the fields of surgical robotics and biomedical engineering, it is likely that we will see the emergence of new, less invasive techniques that could revolutionize treatment in orthopedic neurosurgery. The growing use of data-driven approaches and artificial intelligence could also improve surgical outcomes by enabling more precise planning of interventions.

Practical work on Navigated Surgery in Implantology

Introduction to Computer-Assisted Surgery in Implantology

Navigated surgery in implantology is an innovative technique that uses navigation systems to guide the placement of dental implants with increased precision. This method relies on the integration of advanced technologies such as 3D imaging, computer modeling and surgical navigation devices. The main aim is to improve clinical results while reducing the risk of complications.

Practical work objectives

- **Understanding of Fundamental Concepts**: Students should acquire a thorough understanding of the basic principles of navigated surgery, including the imaging techniques used (such as computed tomography) and their application in implantology.

- **Analysis of Advantages and Disadvantages**: Students will be asked to assess the potential advantages of this approach over traditional methods, as well as the challenges associated with its use.

- **Case Study Practice**: Students will be asked to examine a clinical case where navigated surgery has been used for the placement of dental implants. They will be asked to analyze the results obtained and discuss the clinical implications.

- **Virtual Simulation**: Use simulation software to plan an implant case using navigated surgery. This includes selecting implant sites, evaluating surrounding anatomical structures and creating a detailed surgical plan.

- **Ethical and Professional Discussion**: Students will be asked to reflect on the ethical considerations surrounding the use of advanced technologies in dentistry, including informed consent and equitable access to care.

Methodology

- **Theoretical lectures**: Theoretical sessions will be organized to introduce key concepts.
- **Practical workshops**: Practical workshops will enable students to use surgical planning software.
- **Discussion groups**: Small-group discussions will encourage the exchange of ideas on the case studies presented.
- **Final Evaluation**: A final presentation where each student or group will present their findings on a specific clinical case.

Conclusion

Navigated surgery represents a significant advance in the field of implantology, offering promising possibilities for improving precision and reducing the risks associated with dental implant placement. This practical work aims to prepare students to integrate these technologies into their future professional practice.

Chapter 9: Laser surgery

Technological innovations in ophthalmic laser surgery have evolved significantly over the last few decades, transforming clinical practices and improving patient outcomes. These advances include various types of lasers used to treat ocular conditions such as myopia, hyperopia, astigmatism and other refractive disorders. The most commonly used laser surgery techniques include laser-assisted in situ keratomileusis (LASIK), refractive photokeratectomy (PRK) and the femtosecond laser.

Technological Innovations

- **Excimer laser**: The excimer laser is a type of ultraviolet laser used to reshape the cornea with great precision. It is used in LASIK and PRK procedures to correct refractive errors. The technology has evolved to include eye-tracking systems that adjust the treatment in real time, increasing safety and efficiency.

- **Femtosecond laser**: This type of laser uses ultrashort pulses to create precise cuts in corneal tissue without direct contact. This has improved the precision of corneal incisions and paved the way for less invasive surgical techniques.

- **Eye Tracking Technologies**: Modern systems incorporate advanced technologies such as 3D imaging and dynamic eye movement tracking, enabling surgeons to make more precise corrections during procedures.

- **Glaucoma Laser Surgery**: Innovations in the field of glaucoma, such as selective laser trabeculoplasty (SLT), have been developed to reduce intraocular pressure with fewer side effects than traditional drug treatments.

- **Therapeutic applications**: In addition to refractive correction, lasers are also used in the treatment of retinal diseases such as age-related macular degeneration (AMD) and retinopathic diabetes, offering a targeted approach to preserving vision.

Clinical Practices

Integrating these technologies into clinical practice requires in-depth training for ophthalmologists to master these advanced tools. In addition, it is essential to carefully assess each patient to determine the appropriate surgical approach for their specific condition.

Clinical studies continue to evaluate the long-term efficacy and safety of laser procedures, helping to establish evidence-based protocols that guide therapeutic decisions.

1. Principles of medical lasers

a) Dioxide lasers

Carbon dioxide (CO2) lasers are optical devices that use carbon dioxide as the active medium to produce a laser beam. They are widely used in various industrial, medical and scientific applications due to their efficiency, power and the specific wavelength they emit, generally around 10.6 micrometers. This wavelength is particularly effective for interacting with organic materials, and is therefore highly prized in the fields of cutting, welding and engraving.

Operating principles

The carbon dioxide laser operates on the principle of stimulated emission. In this type of laser, a gas mixture containing mainly CO2, as well as other gases such as nitrogen (N2) and helium (He), is excited by an external energy source, often an electric current. When CO2 molecules are excited, they move to a higher energy state. On returning to their ground state, these molecules emit photons in the process of stimulated emission. These photons can then be amplified by successive reflections between two mirrors placed at the ends of the laser tube.

Applications

1. **Industry**: CO2 lasers are used for cutting and welding metals and plastics, thanks to their ability to generate intense heat concentrated over a small area.

2. **Medicine**: In the medical field, these lasers are used for surgical procedures such as dermatology (treatment of scars and skin lesions) and eye surgery (such as laser-assisted in situ keratomileusis - LASIK).

3. **Scientific research**: CO2 lasers are also used in various scientific instruments for precise measurements or as light sources in experiments.

4. **Spectroscopy**: Thanks to their unique properties, they play a crucial role in spectroscopic analysis, where they can excite certain molecules to study their characteristics.

5. **Optical communication**: Although less common than other types of lasers in this field, CO2 lasers can also be used in certain optical communication applications.

Benefits

Carbon dioxide lasers offer several advantages:

- **Energy efficiency**: They are highly efficient compared with other types of laser.
- **Long service life**: Their components tend to have a longer service life.

- **Ability to handle a variety of materials**: They can interact effectively with different types of material.

Disadvantages : However, there are also some disadvantages:

- **High initial cost**: Installation may require a substantial investment.
- **Size and weight**: CO2 systems can be bulkier than some other types of laser.
- **Safety**: Like all powerful lasers, they require strict safety precautions to prevent injury.

b) Erbium lasers

Erbium lasers, often referred to as Er:YAG (erbium-doped Yttrium Aluminium Garnet) lasers, are optical devices that emit coherent light in the infrared region of the electromagnetic spectrum. They are widely used in a variety of fields, including medicine, dentistry, aesthetics and industrial applications. The importance of these lasers lies in their ability to interact with biological tissues and materials in a precise and controlled manner.

Operating principles

The erbium laser works on the principle of stimulated emission. Erbium is a rare chemical element which, when excited by an external energy source (such as a flashlamp or diode laser), emits photons at a specific wavelength, usually around 2940 nm. This wavelength is particularly effective at being absorbed by water, making erbium lasers very useful for applications where water is a major component of the targeted tissue.

Medical applications

1. **Dermatological surgery**: erbium lasers are used for skin resurfacing, removing superficial layers of damaged skin while minimizing damage to

surrounding tissue. This promotes rapid healing and reduces the risk of scarring.

2. **Dentistry**: In the dental field, these lasers enable less invasive procedures for tooth decay and gum treatment. Their precision helps preserve more healthy tissue.

3. **Orthopedic surgery**: erbium lasers are also used to treat certain orthopedic conditions, thanks to their ability to cut or vaporize bone or cartilage tissue with precision.

4. **Aesthetics**: In cosmetics, they are used to reduce wrinkles and improve skin texture.

Advantages: The advantages of erbium lasers include :

- **Precision**: They enable precise incision without damaging adjacent tissue.
- **Fewer side effects**: Compared to other types of laser, they have fewer side effects, such as inflammation.
- **Rapid recovery**: Patients often benefit from a shorter recovery period.

Limitations: However, there are also certain limitations:

- **High cost**: Laser equipment can be expensive.
- **Need for specialized training**: Safe, effective use requires proper training to avoid complications.

c) Dye lasers

Pulsed dye lasers are optical devices that use organic dyes as the active medium to produce a laser beam. They are distinguished by their ability to emit a wide range of wavelengths, making them particularly useful in a variety of scientific and industrial applications. In-depth, practical studies of these lasers involve several aspects, including their design, operation, applications and the challenges associated with their use.

1. Design and operation of pulsed dye lasers

Pulsed dye lasers operate on the principle of stimulated emission of radiation. The active medium, consisting of dye molecules dissolved in a solvent, is excited by an external energy source, usually a pumping laser. This excitation process enables the dye molecules to reach a high-energy state. When they return to their ground state, they emit photons that can be amplified by feedback in a resonant cavity.

The design of a pulsed dye laser involves the appropriate selection of the dye, the configuration of the optical system (including mirrors and amplifying medium), and the choice of the pumping system. Dye lasers can be configured to operate in either continuous or pulsed mode, the latter being particularly popular for its applications in spectroscopy and imaging.

2. Pulsed dye laser applications : The applications of pulsed dye lasers are varied and cover several fields:

- **Spectroscopy**: Thanks to their ability to emit different wavelengths, these lasers are used to analyze the chemical composition of substances.
- **Biological imaging**: in the medical field, they enable high-resolution imaging of biological tissues.
- **Laser treatment** : Used in certain dermatological procedures to treat skin lesions.
- **Fundamental research**: They play a crucial role in the study of quantum phenomena and light-matter interactions.

3. Challenges associated with pulsed dye lasers: Despite their advantages, pulsed dye lasers present certain challenges:

- **Stability of active medium**: Organic colorants can degrade over time or under the effect of intense light.
- **System complexity**: The need for sophisticated pumping and thermal management equipment can make these systems costly and difficult to maintain.
- **Spectral limitations**: Although they have a wide range of available wavelengths, each type of laser has its own limitations in terms of power and efficiency.

d) **ND:YAG lasers**

Neodymium-doped yttrium aluminum garnet (Nd:YAG) crystal lasers are laser devices widely used in a variety of fields, including medicine, industry and scientific research. This type of laser is particularly appreciated for its ability to produce specific wavelengths, making it effective for a variety of applications.

Operating principles

The Nd:YAG laser works on the principle of stimulated emission of radiation. The YAG (Yttrium Aluminium Garnet) crystal is doped with neodymium ions (Nd^{3+}), which act as the laser's active atoms. When an external energy source excites these ions, they change to a higher energy state. On returning to their ground state, these ions emit photons, producing a coherent laser beam.

The main wavelength emitted by the Nd:YAG laser is 1064 nm in the near infrared. This wavelength is particularly useful for its ability to penetrate biological tissue, making it a preferred choice for medical applications such as laser surgery and treatment of skin lesions.

Medical applications

In the medical field, Nd:YAG lasers are used for a variety of surgical procedures, including lithotripsy (fragmentation of kidney stones), photocoagulation and treatment of varicose veins. Their ability to precisely target tissue while minimizing damage to surrounding tissue makes them a valuable tool for surgeons.

In dermatology, these lasers are used to treat conditions such as pigmentation spots and scars. The ability of the Nd:YAG laser to penetrate deep into the skin enables effective stimulation of collagen, promoting tissue regeneration.

Industrial applications

Nd:YAG lasers are also used in industry for applications such as welding, cutting and marking. Their high power and precision enable efficient handling of metallic and non-metallic materials. In the automotive industry, for example, these lasers are used to weld parts with great precision, without affecting the mechanical properties of the material.

Advantages and disadvantages

The advantages of the Nd:YAG laser include its robustness, durability and ability to operate in a variety of environmental conditions. However, it also has certain drawbacks, such as its relatively high cost compared with other types of laser, and the need for adequate cooling during prolonged use.

e) Alexandrite lasers

Alexandrite lasers are optical devices that use an Alexandrite crystal as the active medium for laser light generation. This type of laser is particularly popular in various fields, including dermatology, aesthetics and industry. Alexandrite is a rare mineral with a unique property: its ability to change color depending on illumination, making it a fascinating material for laser applications.

Operating principles

The Alexandrite laser works on the principle of stimulated emission of radiation. When an Alexandrite crystal is excited by an external energy source (usually a flash lamp), it emits photons in a specific range of wavelengths, mainly around 755 nm, which lies in the near-infrared spectrum. This wavelength is particularly effective at targeting melanin in the skin, making the Alexandrite laser very useful for permanent hair removal treatments and the treatment of pigmented lesions.

Clinical applications

1. **Laser Hair Removal**: The Alexandrite laser is widely used for permanent hair removal thanks to its ability to effectively target hair follicles while minimizing damage to surrounding tissue. It is particularly effective on fair skin with dark hair.

2. **Treatment of vascular lesions**: Thanks to its specific wavelength, the Alexandrite laser can also be used to treat various vascular lesions such as spider veins and telangiectasias.

3. **Skin rejuvenation**: The laser's properties also enable its use in skin rejuvenation, where it helps reduce the appearance of wrinkles and improve overall skin texture.

4. **Tattoos**: Although less common than other types of lasers, the Alexandrite laser can be used to remove certain types of tattoo by targeting specific pigments.

5. **Ophthalmic surgery**: In some cases, the Alexandrite laser has been explored for eye-related surgical applications, although this is less frequent compared to other types of laser used in this field.

Advantages and disadvantages

Alexandrite lasers offer a number of advantages, not least their efficacy on different skin types and their speed of treatment. However, they also require considerable expertise to avoid side effects such as hyperpigmentation or hypopigmentation.

2. Applications in ophthalmology, dermatology and oncology

A. Clinical applications of laser surgery in dermatology

Laser surgery in dermatology is a discipline that has evolved significantly over the last few decades. Lasers are used to treat a variety of skin conditions, from benign lesions to more complex conditions such as melanoma. Clinical applications of lasers in dermatology can be classified into several categories, including skin resurfacing, removal of pigmented lesions, treatment of blood vessels and scar management.

1. Skin resurfacing

Laser skin resurfacing is a technique that uses fractionated or unfractionated lasers to improve skin texture, reduce wrinkles and treat acne scars. Fractional lasers allow specific areas of the skin to be targeted while leaving other areas untouched, promoting faster healing and reducing the risk of side effects.

2. Removal of Pigmented Lesions

Pulsed dye lasers and Q-switched lasers are commonly used to treat pigmented lesions such as age spots, solar lentigines and tattoos. These lasers work by specifically targeting melanin in the skin, enabling selective destruction without damaging surrounding tissue.

3. Blood vessel treatment

Vascular lasers, such as the pulsed dye laser and the Nd:YAG laser, are effective in treating various vascular conditions such as telangiectasias (dilated blood vessels) and angiomas. These treatments work by photocoagulation, where laser energy causes blood to coagulate in the targeted vessels, leading to their gradual disappearance.

4. Scar Management

Hypertrophic and keloid scars can also be successfully treated by laser. Laser treatment can help reduce the appearance of these scars by reshaping the underlying collagen and improving skin elasticity.

5. Advantages and disadvantages of laser surgery in dermatology

Laser surgery has become a widely used treatment method in dermatology, offering a variety of applications from skin rejuvenation to the removal of pigmented lesions and scars. Dermatological lasers work by emitting concentrated beams of light that specifically target skin tissue, enabling a variety of problems to be treated without damaging surrounding tissue. This technology has its advantages and disadvantages, which we will explore in depth.

Advantages of laser surgery in dermatology

1. **Precision**: One of the main advantages of laser surgery is its ability to precisely target affected areas. Lasers can be set to treat specific layers of skin, minimizing damage to adjacent healthy tissue.

2. **Less discomfort**: Compared to traditional surgical methods, laser treatment can result in less pain and discomfort post surgery. Many patients report faster recovery with fewer side effects.

3. **Improved aesthetic results**: Laser treatments can improve skin appearance by reducing wrinkles, acne scars and pigment spots. Results are often visible after a single session, although several treatments may be required to achieve optimal effect.

4. **Versatility**: Laser surgery can treat a wide range of dermatological conditions, including but not limited to psoriasis, eczema, warts, and even some forms of skin cancer.

5. **Less bleeding**: Lasers also coagulate blood vessels during treatment, reducing the risk of bleeding compared to conventional surgical techniques.

Disadvantages of laser surgery in dermatology

1. **High cost**: The cost of laser treatments can be prohibitive for some patients. The high cost of equipment and the potential need for several sessions can make these treatments inaccessible to a wide audience.

2. **Risks of side effects**: Although generally considered safe, laser surgery carries certain risks, such as hyperpigmentation or hypopigmentation (change in skin color), potential infections and scarring.

3. **Variable downtime**: Depending on the type of treatment performed, some patients may require significant downtime to allow their skin to heal properly after treatment.

4. **Skill required**: The success of the treatment is highly dependent on the skill of the practitioner using the laser. Incorrect use can lead to unsatisfactory results or even aggravate the condition being treated.

5. **Limitations in certain clinical cases**: Not all types of skin lesions respond well to laser treatment; some conditions may require other forms of medical or surgical intervention.

B. <u>Laser surgery applications in oncology</u>

Laser surgery is a technique that uses concentrated beams of light to perform surgical procedures. In oncology, this method has gained in popularity thanks to its potential advantages over traditional surgical techniques. Laser applications in oncology include tumor ablation, reduction of tumor size, and palliative treatment to relieve symptoms associated with advanced cancers.

Principles of Laser Surgery

Laser surgery is based on the principle of selective photothermolysis, where a laser beam is directed at the targeted tissue. The laser can be adjusted to specifically target cancer cells while minimizing damage to surrounding healthy tissue. Types of lasers used in oncology include the CO2 laser, the Nd:YAG (neodymium-doped yttrium-aluminum-garnet) laser, and the argon laser.

Operating principles of laser surgery in oncology

Laser surgery in oncology is a technique that uses concentrated beams of light to treat cancerous tumors. This method offers several advantages over traditional surgical techniques, including reduced pain, shorter recovery times and fewer post-operative complications. Lasers can be used to destroy cancer cells, reduce the size of tumors prior to more invasive surgery, or even to perform biopsies.

Operating principles

1. **Types of lasers**: There are several types of lasers used in oncology, each with specific wavelengths adapted to different types of tissue. CO2 lasers, for example, are often used for superficial tumors, as they are efficiently absorbed by water in the tissue.

2. **Mechanism of action**: The fundamental principle behind laser surgery is the selective absorption of the laser beam by the target tissue. When the laser is directed at a tumor, light energy is converted into heat, resulting in

the thermal destruction of cancer cells without significantly damaging surrounding tissue.

3. **Clinical applications**: Laser surgery is used in a variety of oncological settings, including the treatment of lung cancer, skin cancer and ENT (ear, nose and throat) cancers. It can be used to excise tumor lesions or to relieve obstructions caused by tumors.

4. **Advantages and disadvantages**:

Laser surgery in oncology is a technique that has gained in popularity due to its many advantages over traditional surgical methods. This approach uses concentrated beams of light to destroy cancer cells, offering several notable benefits.

Advantages of Laser Surgery in Oncology

a) **Greater precision**: Laser surgery enables greater precision in the ablation of tumor tissue. Lasers can target cancer cells with great accuracy, minimizing damage to surrounding healthy tissue. This is particularly important in delicate areas such as the brain or reproductive organs.

b) **Less invasive**: Compared to traditional surgical techniques, laser surgery is generally less invasive. It often requires smaller incisions, which reduces trauma to the patient's body and promotes faster recovery.

c) **Reduced pain and bleeding**: The use of lasers can lead to less bleeding during surgery, as the laser beam coagulates blood vessels as it cuts. This translates into less post-operative pain and a reduced need for painkillers.

d) **Rapid recovery**: Patients undergoing laser surgery tend to have shorter recovery times than those who have undergone traditional surgery. This means they can return to their daily activities more quickly, improving their quality of life after the procedure.

e) **Less scarring**: Since laser surgery often requires smaller incisions, this leads to less visible scarring compared to conventional surgical methods involving larger incisions.

f) **Varied applications**: Laser surgery can be used to treat various types of cancer, including those affecting the skin, lungs, and even some gynecological cancers. Its versatility makes it a valuable tool in the cancer treatment arsenal.

g) **Fewer infections**: Because of the less invasive aspect and the smaller incisions, there is also a reduced risk of post-operative infection compared to traditional surgical procedures.

5. **Limits and considerations of laser surgery in oncology**

Laser surgery in oncology is a technique that uses concentrated beams of light to treat tumors. This method offers several advantages over traditional surgical techniques, including reduced bleeding, less post-operative pain, and faster recovery time. However, it also has important limitations and considerations that need to be taken into account.

Limits of laser surgery

a) **Limited indications**: Not all tumor types are suitable for laser treatment. For example, very large tumors or those located in hard-to-reach areas may require other surgical approaches.

b) **Specialized training required**: Handling lasers requires specific training; not all surgeons are qualified to perform these procedures.

c) **High costs**: Laser equipment can be expensive to acquire and maintain, which may limit its use in some medical facilities.

Clinical considerations

a) **Pre-operative assessment**: Careful evaluation is essential to determine whether a patient is a good candidate for laser surgery.

b) **Post-operative follow-up**: Patients should be followed closely after the procedure to monitor any potential complications or tumor recurrence.

c) **Ongoing research**: Although research into the use of lasers in oncology is promising, much remains to be learned about their long-term effects and effectiveness compared to conventional treatments.

6. Future prospects for laser surgery in oncology

Laser surgery in oncology represents a significant advance in cancer treatment, offering less invasive alternatives to traditional surgical methods. The use of lasers in oncology is based on physical and biological principles that enable precise targeting of tumor tissue while minimizing damage to surrounding healthy tissue.

Future prospects

The future of laser surgery in oncology looks promising thanks to several technological developments:

- **Fiber-optic laser**: This technology provides better access to hard-to-reach areas and greater flexibility during procedures.
- **Combination therapies**: Integrating laser therapy with other therapeutic modalities such as immunotherapy or chemotherapy could improve overall treatment efficacy.

- **Development of new types of lasers**: Research continues into the use of new types of lasers that could offer even greater advantages in terms of efficiency and safety.

Challenges and considerations: Despite its advantages, laser surgery also presents certain challenges:

- **High cost**: Laser equipment can be expensive, limiting its availability in some medical institutions.
- **Specialized training required**: Surgeons need specific training to use these technologies effectively.
- **Anatomical limitations**: In some cases, the patient's anatomy may make it difficult to access tumors with a laser beam.

Practical Work on Myopia Correction by Laser Surgery

Introduction

Myopia, or blurred vision at a distance, is a common visual disorder affecting millions of people worldwide. Laser surgery, including laser-assisted in situ keratomileusis (LASIK) and refractive photokeratectomy (PRK), are popular methods of correcting this problem. This practical work aims to explore the principles, techniques, benefits and risks associated with these procedures.

Practical work objectives

1. **Understanding myopia**: Define myopia and explain its physiological mechanism.
2. **Explore Surgical Techniques**: Study the different laser surgical techniques used to correct myopia.

3. **Analyze the advantages and disadvantages**: Evaluate the benefits and risks associated with these interventions.
4. **Post-operative considerations**: Discuss the post-operative care required after laser surgery.
5. **Case studies**: Analyze real-life case studies to understand the impact of these procedures on patients' quality of life.

Part 1: Understanding Myopia

Myopia occurs when the eyeball is too long or the cornea has too pronounced a curvature, preventing light from reaching the retina properly. This results in blurred vision of distant objects.

Part 2: Surgical techniques

2.1 Laser-assisted in situ keratomileusis (LASIK)

LASIK is one of the most common procedures for correcting myopia. It involves creating a flap in the cornea, then using an excimer laser to reshape the underlying corneal tissue to enable better focusing of the light on the retina.

2.2 Refractive photokeratectomy (PRK)

PRK is another technique that involves the removal of corneal tissue without creating a flap. This method may be preferable for certain patients with insufficient corneal thickness.

Part 3: Advantages and disadvantages

Advantages include rapid recovery, less dependence on glasses or contact lenses, and a significant improvement in vision. However, there are also risks such as post-operative discomfort, risk of infection and unsatisfactory visual results.

Part 4: Post-operative considerations

After laser surgery, it's crucial that patients follow certain recommendations such as using prescribed eye drops, avoiding strenuous physical activity for a few weeks and attending follow-up appointments with their ophthalmologist.

Part 5: Case studies

Analysis of clinical studies shows that patient satisfaction after laser surgery is generally high, but it is essential to evaluate each case individually, taking into account factors such as patient age and degree of myopia.

Conclusion

Surgical laser correction offers an effective solution for treating myopia in many individuals. However, it is imperative that every patient is fully informed about the options available, as well as the potential risks, before undertaking this procedure.

Stimulated emission of medical laser principle

Stimulated emission is a fundamental phenomenon underlying the operation of lasers, including medical lasers. The process was first theorized by Albert Einstein in 1917, but it was only with the technological development of the 20th century that practical applications emerged, particularly in the medical field.

Principle of Stimulated Emission

Stimulated emission occurs when photons interact with atoms or molecules in an excited state. When a photon of a certain wavelength encounters an excited atom, it can cause a second photon to be emitted. This new photon is coherent with the first, meaning it has the same phase, frequency and direction. This mechanism is the basis of laser light generation.

Medical laser applications: Medical lasers are used in a variety of clinical applications, from surgery to dermatology. Common types of medical lasers include:

- **Carbon dioxide (CO_2) lasers**: Used primarily for dermatological and cosmetic surgery, these lasers enable precise incisions and minimize damage to surrounding tissue.

- **YAG (Yttrium-Aluminium-Garnet) lasers**: These lasers are often used to treat kidney stones and perform ophthalmic procedures such as capsulotomy.

- **Dye lasers**: Used to treat various skin conditions such as vascular and pigmented lesions.

- **Fiber lasers**: Increasingly popular for their flexibility and efficiency, they are used in a variety of surgical procedures.

- **Argon lasers**: often used in ophthalmology to treat certain retinal diseases.

Underlying physical mechanisms : The operation of medical lasers is based on several physical principles:

- **Inverted population**: For a laser to work, you need to create an inverted population where more atoms or molecules are in an excited state than in the ground state.

- **Laser cavity** : The light emitted is amplified by reflection between two mirrors placed at the ends of an optical cavity.

- **Wavelength control**: Modern devices allow precise control of laser wavelength, which is crucial for targeting specific tissues without damaging surrounding tissue.

Clinical practices: Practitioners need to be trained not only in the technical use of lasers, but also in the biological and physiological implications of their use. This includes:

- Understanding the interactions between lasers and biological tissues.
- Assessment of potential risks such as burns or scars.
- Appropriate application depending on the type of tissue targeted (e.g. skin vs. connective tissue).

The inverted population of the medical laser principle

The principle of inverted population is fundamental to the operation of lasers, including medical lasers. This concept is based on the need to have a greater number of atoms or molecules in an excited state than in a ground state. This enables the excited atoms to be stimulated to emit coherent photons, which is essential for generating the laser beam.

1. Inverse Population Principle

Inverse population occurs when the energy levels of a quantum system are unconventionally occupied, i.e. more atoms are in an excited state than in the ground state. To achieve this condition, an external energy source is usually required, often referred to as "pumping". In the medical context, this can be achieved by a variety of methods, such as optical or electrical excitation.

2. Medical applications of lasers

Medical lasers use the inverted population principle to treat a variety of medical conditions. For example, carbon dioxide (CO2) and neodymium-yttrium-aluminum-garnet (Nd:YAG) lasers are commonly used in dermatology and surgery. These devices enable precise procedures with minimal damage to surrounding tissue, thanks to their ability to deliver concentrated energy to a small area.

3. Types of medical lasers: There are several types of medical lasers that exploit the principle of inverted population:

- **CO2 laser**: Mainly used for dermatological and cosmetic surgery.
- **Nd:YAG laser**: Used to treat varicose veins and certain forms of cancer.
- **Er:YAG laser**: Used for dental and dermatological procedures.
- **Dye laser** : Used to treat vascular and pigmented lesions.

Each type has its own characteristics in terms of wavelength, penetration depth and efficacy, depending on the clinical application.

4. Mechanisms of Action: The mechanisms by which these lasers act include :

- **Selective photothermolysis**: Specific targeting of abnormal tissue without damaging healthy tissue.
- **Collagen stimulation**: Promotes tissue regeneration after treatment.

- **Evaporation or ablation**: Removes superficial layers of skin or other tissue.

5. Advantages and limitations : Advantages of medical lasers include:

- Greater precision
- Fewer side effects
- Fast recovery

However, there are also limitations such as :

- High cost
- Need for specialized training
- Potential risks if misused

The coherence and mono chromaticity of the medical laser principle

Coherence

Laser coherence refers to the ability of photons emitted by the laser to maintain a constant phase relationship over a certain distance. This is crucial in medical applications where precision is paramount. For example, in laser treatments to remove tumors or treat skin lesions, coherence enables precise targeting of tissue without damaging surrounding tissue. Coherence can be classified into two types: temporal coherence and spatial coherence.

- **Temporal coherence**: This refers to the length of time a light beam remains correlated over time. A laser with high temporal coherence can produce very short pulses that are ideal for delicate surgical procedures.

- **Spatial coherence**: This concerns the uniformity of the beam's phase across its cross-section. Good spatial coherence is necessary to obtain a narrow beam that can be precisely focused.

Monochromaticity

The monochromaticity of a laser indicates that the beam emitted has a single or very narrow wavelength. This is particularly important in medical treatments, as different wavelengths interact differently with biological tissues. For example:

- Wavelength-specific lasers can target particular chromophores in the skin, such as melanin or hemoglobin, enabling effective treatment while minimizing damage to surrounding tissue.

- The ability to choose a precise wavelength also enables doctors to tailor treatments to the patient's specific needs.

Clinical applications: The properties of coherence and monochromaticity make medical lasers extremely useful in a number of areas:

- **Eye surgery**: excimer lasers are used to correct vision by precisely reshaping the cornea.

- **Dermatology**: Pulsed dye lasers effectively treat vascular and pigmented lesions.

- **Oncology**: Lasers can be used to destroy cancer cells with minimal effect on surrounding healthy tissue.

- **Dentistry**: Lasers enable less invasive procedures with less post-operative pain.

- **Physical therapies**: Use of lasers to relieve pain and promote healing.

The principle of medical laser surgery

The fundamental principle of the laser (acronym for "Light Amplification by Stimulated Emission of Radiation") is based on the stimulated emission of photons, resulting in a coherent, monochromatic and directional beam of light. This technology has revolutionized several medical fields, including dermatology, ophthalmology and general surgery.

Basic principles of medical lasers

- **Laser physics**: Lasers work on the principle of stimulated emission. When an atom or molecule is excited by an external energy source, it can emit a photon when it returns to a lower energy state. In an amplifying environment, these photons can stimulate other atoms to emit even more photons, creating light amplification.

- **Types of lasers**: There are several types of lasers used in medicine, each with specific characteristics adapted to different applications:
  - **CO2 laser**: Used mainly for dermatological and surgical procedures, due to its ability to cut tissue with precision.
  - **Nd:YAG laser**: Used for in-depth treatments such as lithotripsy and certain ophthalmic procedures.
  - **Er:YAG laser**: Preferred for superficial treatments such as skin resurfacing.

1. **Clinical applications**:

   - **Ophthalmic surgery**: Laser-assisted in situ keratomileusis (LASIK) is a popular procedure for correcting vision.
   - **Dermatology**: Lasers are used to treat skin lesions such as acne scars and pigment spots.
   - **Oncology surgery**: Lasers can eliminate tumors with less damage to surrounding tissue.

2. **Advantages and disadvantages**:

- Benefits include reduced bleeding, rapid recovery and less post-operative pain.
- However, there are also potential drawbacks, such as the risk of thermal burns or side effects related to the skin or eyes.

3. **Training and Clinical Practice**: Training in laser surgery requires a thorough understanding of the underlying physical principles as well as practical expertise in the use of laser devices. This includes not only technical handling, but also the management of potential complications.

Practical work: Light in eye surgery and the usefulness of the Femtosecond Laser

Introduction

Light plays a crucial role in eye surgery, thanks in particular to the use of advanced technologies such as the femtosecond laser. This practical work aims to explore the fundamental principles of light as a surgical tool, as well as the specific applications of the femtosecond laser in various ophthalmic procedures.

1. Principles of Light

Light is a form of electromagnetic energy that propagates in the form of waves. In the context of eye surgery, it is essential to understand the properties of light, such as :

- **Refraction**: The deflection of light rays as they pass from one medium to another.
- **Diffraction**: The phenomenon whereby light waves bend around obstacles.
- **Interference**: The superposition of two light waves, which can increase or decrease their intensity.

These principles are fundamental to understanding how surgical instruments use light to visualize and treat ocular structures.

2. The Femtosecond Laser

The femtosecond laser is a revolutionary technology that uses ultra-short pulses (in the femtosecond range) to make precise incisions in ocular tissue. Here are some key features:

- **Precision**: femtosecond lasers enable extremely precise incisions, minimizing damage to surrounding tissue.
- **Safety**: Thanks to their ability to target specific tissue layers, these lasers reduce the risk of post-operative complications.
- **Applications**: Used in a variety of procedures such as refractive surgery (LASIK), cataract and even some retinal procedures.

3. Clinical applications: Clinical applications of the femtosecond laser include :

- **Refractive surgery**: Correction of refractive errors such as myopia, hyperopia and astigmatism.
- **Cataract surgery**: Facilitates extraction of the opacified lens with greater precision.

- **Creation of corneal flaps**: Essential for LASIK procedures, where a corneal flap is created prior to laser reshaping.

4. Advantages and disadvantages : Although the femtosecond laser has several advantages, there are also potential disadvantages:

Advantages :

- Less invasive than traditional techniques.
- Faster recovery for patients.

Disadvantages :

- High cost of equipment.
- Need for specialized training for surgeons.

Conclusion

The integration of light and laser technologies into eye surgery has transformed this medical specialty. The femtosecond laser represents a significant advance, offering precision and safety to patients while improving clinical outcomes.

C. Ophthalmology in laser surgery

The applications of laser surgery in ophthalmology have evolved significantly over the last few decades, offering considerable benefits while presenting certain risks. This in-depth analysis focuses on the main types of laser procedures used in ophthalmology, the benefits associated with these techniques, and the potential complications that can arise.

Advantages of laser surgery applications in ophthalmology

- **Precision and control**: lasers enable exceptional surgical precision. For example, in refractive surgery such as LASIK (Laser-Assisted In Situ Keratomileusis), the excimer laser can reshape the cornea with great accuracy, improving vision without the need for implants or lenses.

- **Rapid recovery**: Patients undergoing laser procedures often enjoy a faster recovery than with traditional surgical methods. This is due to the minimal invasiveness of these techniques, which reduces healing time and enables a rapid return to daily activities.

- **Less post-operative pain**: Laser procedures are generally associated with less post-operative pain. Laser technology reduces tissue trauma, which in turn reduces the discomfort felt by the patient after the procedure.

- **Long-lasting results**: Many laser procedures offer long-lasting, stable results over time. For example, LASIK vision correction has shown high rates of long-term patient satisfaction.

- **A wide range of applications**: Lasers are used to treat a variety of eye conditions, such as glaucoma (with selective laser treatment), cataracts (with laser-assisted phacoemulsification) and retinal diseases (such as photocoagulation).

Risks associated with laser surgery applications

- **Potential complications**: Although rare, certain complications may arise after laser surgery. These include problems such as hypercorrection or hypocorrection of vision, as well as side effects such as dry eyes or night-time glare.

- **Eligibility limitations**: Not all patients are candidates for laser surgery. Factors such as insufficient corneal thickness or certain pre-existing eye diseases may limit the use of the laser.

- **High cost**: Laser procedures can be expensive and are not always covered by health insurance, which can be an obstacle for some patients.

- **Technology-related risks**: As with any medical technology, there is a risk of human or technical error when using laser equipment, which could lead to undesirable results.

- **Rapid technological evolution**: The constant evolution of laser technologies can make certain techniques rapidly obsolete or less effective than new, emerging methods.

Laser surgery applications in ophthalmology

Lasers are used to modify ocular tissues with extreme precision, offering effective solutions for problems such as myopia, hyperopia, astigmatism and other retinal pathologies.

1. Types of lasers used in ophthalmology: The main types of lasers used in ophthalmology include :

- **Excimer laser**: mainly used for refractive surgery such as LASIK (Laser-Assisted In Situ Keratomileusis) and PRK (Photorefractive Keratectomy). This type of laser reshapes the cornea to correct refractive errors.
- **YAG laser (Yttrium-Aluminium-Garnet)**: Used to perform post-operative capsulotomies after cataract surgery, eliminating the blur caused by opacification of the lens capsule.
- **Argon laser**: Used to treat retinal diseases such as diabetic retinopathy and retinal detachment. It coagulates abnormal blood vessels.

2. Clinical applications: The clinical applications of lasers in ophthalmology are varied:

- **Refractive surgery**: Correcting visual defects is one of the most common applications. Procedures such as LASIK and PRK have revolutionized the treatment of visual disorders, enabling millions of patients to achieve clear vision without glasses or contacts.

- **Glaucoma treatment**: Lasers can be used to reduce intraocular pressure in glaucoma patients. Laser trabeculoplasty is a common method for improving intraocular fluid flow.

- **Cataract surgery**: The use of femtosecond lasers in cataract surgery enables greater precision during corneal incision and lens fragmentation.

Technological innovations in ophthalmic laser surgery

Laser surgery in ophthalmology has evolved significantly over the last few decades, transforming the landscape of eye disease treatment. Technological innovations in this field have improved the precision, safety and efficiency of surgical procedures. Here is a detailed analysis of the main advances and their clinical applications.

1. Introduction to laser surgery in ophthalmology

Laser surgery has become an essential tool in the treatment of a variety of eye conditions, including myopia, hyperopia, astigmatism and cataracts. Lasers used in ophthalmology include the excimer laser for vision correction and the YAG laser for cataract treatment.

2. Types of lasers used

- **Excimer laser**: used primarily for laser-assisted in situ keratomileusis (LASIK) and refractive photokeratectomy (PRK) procedures. This type of laser precisely removes corneal layers to modify the curvature of the cornea.

- **Femtosecond laser**: A recent innovation enabling greater precision in corneal incisions. It is used in LASIK procedures to create a bladeless corneal flap, reducing the risk of complications.

- **YAG laser**: Used to treat secondary cataracts by performing a posterior capsulotomy, enabling patients who have undergone initial cataract surgery to regain their visual acuity.

3. Advantages of laser technologies : Technological innovations bring several advantages:

- **Greater precision**: Lasers enable more precise interventions than traditional surgical methods.
- **Rapid recovery**: Patients often enjoy a faster recovery with less post-operative discomfort.
- **Fewer side effects**: Laser technology reduces the risk of infections and other complications associated with conventional surgical techniques.

4. Clinical applications: The clinical applications of lasers in ophthalmology are vast:

- Refractive correction (LASIK, PRK)
- Glaucoma treatment (selective laser)
- Cataract surgery
- Treatment of retinal diseases (photocoagulation)

5. Future prospects

The future of laser surgery in ophthalmology looks bright with the continued emergence of new technologies such as artificial intelligence to further improve surgical results and personalize treatments to individual patient needs.

Laser-assisted in situ keratomileusis

Laser-assisted in situ keratomileusis (LASIK) is a refractive surgical procedure that has revolutionized the treatment of refractive errors such as myopia, hyperopia and astigmatism. This technique uses a laser to reshape the cornea, enabling a significant improvement in vision without the need for glasses or contact lenses.

History and development

The development of LASIK dates back to the 1980s, with the first research into the excimer laser, which enabled precise modification of the cornea. The combination of a corneal incision to create a flap and corneal reshaping using an excimer laser was introduced as an effective method for correcting visual defects.

Methodology: The LASIK procedure consists of several stages:

- **Preparation**: The patient undergoes a complete eye examination to assess ocular health and determine suitability for surgery.

- **Flap creation**: A microkeratome or femtosecond laser is used to create a flap in the cornea. This flap is then lifted to expose the underlying corneal tissue.

- **Corneal reshaping**: An excimer laser is applied to the exposed surface of the cornea to remove specific layers of corneal tissue, thereby modifying its curvature.

- **Flap closure**: The flap is repositioned without the need for stitches, as it adheres naturally to the cornea.

Advantages and disadvantages

The advantages of LASIK include rapid vision recovery, less post-operative discomfort than other refractive surgical procedures, and predictable results. However, there are also associated risks, such as complications related to the flap incision, visual side effects (such as glare or halos), and in some cases, insufficient or excessive correction.

Clinical studies

Numerous studies have been carried out to assess the efficacy and safety of LASIK. Results generally show that over 90% of patients achieve satisfactory visual acuity after surgery. Ongoing research is needed to monitor long-term effects and improve surgical techniques.

Refractive photokeratectolmy

Refractive photokeratectomy (RPK) is a surgical procedure used to correct refractive errors such as myopia, hyperopia and astigmatism. The technique uses an excimer laser to reshape the cornea, enabling vision to be improved without the need for glasses or contact lenses. In-depth, practical studies of PRK focus on several key aspects: clinical indications, surgical techniques, visual results, potential complications and technological advances.

Clinical indications

PRK is generally indicated for patients with stable refractive errors who do not wish to wear glasses or contacts. Eligibility criteria include a sufficiently thick cornea, a minimum age (often 18), and a stable prescription for at least one year. Patients with certain pre-existing eye conditions may be excluded due to the increased risk of complications.

Operating techniques

The procedure begins with topical anesthesia of the eyes to minimize discomfort. The surgeon then uses a device to remove the corneal epithelium, exposing the underlying corneal tissue. The excimer laser is then precisely applied to remove specific layers of corneal tissue according to the patient's refractive profile. After laser treatment, a bandage can be placed over the eye to promote healing.

Visual results

Studies show that the majority of patients achieve satisfactory vision after PRK. According to several studies, around 90% of patients achieve visual acuity of 20/40 or better, which is considered sufficient for driving without glasses. However, there are individual variations in results depending on factors such as age and initial severity of refractive errors.

Potential complications

Although generally considered safe, PRK involves certain risks. Complications may include prolonged post-operative pain, corneal infection, or problems associated with inappropriate healing. Studies have also documented cases of hypercorrection or hypocorrection requiring additional interventions.

Technological advances

Recent advances in refractive surgery have led to the emergence of new techniques and technologies that further improve results and reduce the risks associated with PRK. For example, the use of advanced imaging enables surgeons to obtain precise topographical maps of the cornea prior to surgery.

Laser treatment for retinal diseases

Retinal diseases are a group of pathological conditions that affect the retina, the light-sensitive layer of tissue at the back of the eye. These include age-related macular degeneration (AMD), retinal diabetes, retinal tears and detachments, and neovascularization. Laser treatment has become an essential method in the management of these conditions, offering solutions that can preserve or improve vision.

1. Principles of laser treatment

Laser treatment uses concentrated light beams to target specific areas of the retina. The two main types of laser used are the argon laser and the YAG (Yttrium-Aluminium-Garnet) laser. The argon laser is often used to coagulate abnormal blood vessels in conditions such as diabetic retinopathy, while the YAG laser is used to treat lens opacities following cataract surgery.

2. Clinical applications

- **Diabetic retinopathy**: Laser treatment can reduce the risk of vision loss by targeting abnormal neovessels that form on the surface of the retina.
- **Age-related macular degeneration**: Laser photocoagulation can be used to treat certain types of exudate or hemorrhage.
- **Retinal detachment**: Laser sclerotherapy can help seal retinal tears and prevent complete detachment.

3. Advanced techniques

More advanced techniques such as photodynamic therapy (PDT) combine the use of a photosensitizing drug with laser treatment to specifically target diseased cells while minimizing damage to surrounding tissue.

4. Efficiency and safety

Studies show that laser treatment is generally safe and effective, but it is not free from potential side effects such as temporary or permanent alterations in vision. Careful evaluation by an ophthalmologist is crucial before initiating treatment.

diseases

Rectinal diseases, which affect the rectum and anal region, can include a variety of conditions ranging from hemorrhoids to anal fissures and polyps. Laser treatment is a modern approach that has gained popularity for some of these conditions due to its potential benefits, such as reduced pain, faster recovery time and fewer complications compared to traditional surgical methods.

List of rectinal diseases

- **Hemorrhoids**: Hemorrhoids are swollen veins in the anal region that can cause pain, itching and bleeding. Laser treatment can be used to coagulate blood vessels to reduce swelling and pain.

- **Anal fissures**: An anal fissure is a tear in the mucous membrane of the anal canal, often caused by the difficult passage of stool. Laser treatment can help reduce inflammation and promote healing while minimizing pain.

- **Rectal polyps**: these are outgrowths on the mucous membrane of the rectum that can be benign or early signs of colorectal cancer. Laser treatment enables these polyps to be removed with precision, while preserving the surrounding healthy tissue.

- **Perineal abscess**: An abscess is an accumulation of pus due to infection. Laser drainage can be used to treat abscesses while reducing tissue trauma.

- **Crohn's disease (affecting the rectum)**: This chronic inflammatory disease can lead to complications such as fistulas or strictures in the rectum. Laser treatments can help treat these complications by reducing inflammation and promoting healing.

Laser treatment modes: Laser treatment for rectinal disease typically uses a concentrated beam of light to target diseased tissue without damaging surrounding healthy tissue. Common techniques include:

- **Laser coagulation**: Used to treat hemorrhoids, this method coagulates blood vessels to stop bleeding.
- **Laser excision**: To remove polyps or excise lesions such as those caused by anal fissures.
- **Laser drainage**: Used to treat abscesses, providing effective drainage with less post-operative pain.
- **CO2 laser**: Often used to vaporize diseased tissue while minimizing the impact on surrounding healthy tissue.

Chapter 10: Custom surgery

Introduction

Personalized surgery, also known as personalized medicine or precision medicine, is a rapidly expanding field that aims to tailor surgical interventions to individual patient characteristics. This approach is based on an in-depth understanding of the genetic, biological and environmental variations that influence a patient's response to surgical treatment. The main aim of personalized surgery is to improve clinical outcomes while minimizing the risks and side effects associated with surgical procedures.

Background and development

Personalized surgery is part of the broader framework of personalized medicine, which has emerged thanks to advances in genomics and biomedical technologies. These advances enable better stratification of patients according to their specific characteristics, which can influence not only the choice of surgical technique, but also the type of anesthesia used, post-operative management and even recommendations for rehabilitation.

Approaches and techniques

Approaches used in personalized surgery include:

1. **Genetic analysis**: Genetic testing can identify specific mutations that predispose a patient to certain diseases or influence their response to certain treatments. For example, in the case of cancer, analysis of tumor biomarkers can guide surgical decisions regarding tumor removal.

2. **Advanced imaging**: Imaging techniques such as functional MRI and CT scans enable precise visualization of anatomical structures and pathologies, facilitating more targeted surgical planning.

3. **3D modeling**: The creation of 3D models based on imaging data enables surgeons to simulate the procedure before it is carried out, which can improve accuracy and reduce complications.

4. **Personalized follow-up**: After the operation, individualized follow-up based on the patient's characteristics can help optimize recovery and prevent complications.

Challenges and prospects

Despite its potential benefits, personalized surgery faces a number of challenges. One of the main obstacles is the high cost associated with the advanced technologies required to implement this approach. In addition, there are still gaps in our understanding of the complex interactions between genetic and environmental factors that influence surgical outcomes.

As we move towards fuller integration of these technologies into clinical practice, it is essential to establish standardized protocols to ensure that all patients benefit equally from advances in personalized surgery.

Conclusion

In short, the study of personalized surgery represents a promising frontier in the medical field. By integrating a patient-centered approach based on solid scientific data, it is possible to significantly improve surgical outcomes while better responding to individual patient needs.

1. Genetic-based preoperative planning

Preoperative planning, which involves risk assessment and patient preparation prior to surgery, can benefit considerably from the integration of genetic information. This enables clinicians to better understand individual susceptibilities to disease, responses to treatment and potential complications.

1. The importance of genetics in preoperative planning

Genetics play a crucial role in determining surgical risk. Genetic variations can influence not only the likelihood of disease, but also how a patient reacts to anesthesia or other drugs administered during and after surgery. For example, certain mutations can affect the metabolism of anesthetics, leading to adverse effects or prolonged recovery.

2. Risk assessment

Preoperative risk assessment is essential to minimize complications. Genetic testing can identify high-risk patients based on their genetic profile. This includes conditions such as bleeding disorders, where genetic evaluation can reveal abnormalities that require special attention during surgery.

Understanding genetic variants in personalized surgery

Personalized surgery, also known as personalized medicine or precision medicine, represents an innovative approach that integrates an individual's genetic information to optimize surgical treatments. This method is based on an understanding of the genetic variants that can influence a patient's response to a specific treatment, including surgical interventions.

1. Understanding genetic variants

Genetic variants are changes in an individual's DNA sequence that can affect various aspects of health, including disease susceptibility, drug response and surgical outcomes. In-depth studies of these variants involve the analysis of nucleotide polymorphisms (SNPs), mutations and other forms of genomic variation. These analyses enable researchers and clinicians to better understand how these differences can influence surgical risk, recovery time and treatment efficacy.

2. Applications in Personalized Surgery

In the context of personalized surgery, genetic information is used to :

- **Patient selection**: Identify those most likely to benefit from a specific surgical intervention.
- **Predicting outcomes**: Assessing how a patient might react to a given procedure based on his or her genetic profile.
- **Adapting surgical techniques**: Modifying surgical approaches based on the patient's genetic characteristics to minimize risk and maximize efficacy.

3. Clinical Studies and Research

Numerous clinical studies have been conducted to explore the impact of genetic variants on various types of surgery, including:

- Oncology surgery, where certain mutations can influence the choice of surgical treatment.
- Orthopedic surgery, where variations in genes linked to bone healing can affect post-operative recovery time.

This research underlines the importance of integrating a DNA-based approach into the surgical decision-making process.

4. Ethical and practical challenges

Despite its potential benefits, the implementation of personalized surgery raises several ethical and practical challenges:

- **Data confidentiality** : The secure management of genetic information is crucial to protecting patient privacy.
- **Unequal access to technologies**: There is a risk that only certain populations will have access to these technological advances, which could exacerbate health inequalities.

5. Future prospects

The future of personalized surgery looks bright with the continuing advance of technologies such as high-throughput sequencing and artificial intelligence. These tools will not only enable a better understanding of genetic variants, but also their integration into standardized surgical protocols.

3. Customized treatment

Personalization of treatment is another key aspect of genetics-based preoperative planning. Using genetic information, doctors can tailor their surgical and anesthetic strategies for each individual patient. For example, if a patient has a mutation associated with an altered response to certain painkillers, the doctor can choose an alternative drug to manage postoperative pain.

Personalizing anesthetic protocols in personalized surgery

The personalization of anesthetic protocols in surgery is a rapidly expanding field that aims to tailor anesthetic care to the specific needs of each patient. This individualized approach is based on a thorough understanding of the physiological, psychological and environmental factors that influence a patient's response to anesthesia.

1. Preoperative assessment

Preoperative assessment is crucial in determining the most appropriate anesthetic protocol. This includes a review of medical history, allergies, current medications and comorbidities. Assessment tools such as ASA (American Society of Anesthesiologists) scores can be used to classify patients according to their general state of health and surgical risk.

2. Pharmacogenomics

Pharmacogenomics plays an essential role in the personalization of anesthetics. It studies how genetic variations affect the response to drugs. For example, some patients may metabolize certain anesthetic agents more quickly or more slowly, which can influence the choice of drug and its dosage.

3. Regional anesthesia techniques

Regional anesthesia techniques, such as peripheral nerve blocks, are often used to reduce postoperative pain and improve functional recovery. The selection of these techniques can be tailored to the type of surgery, the patient's anatomy and personal preferences.

4. Multimodal anesthesia

Multimodal anesthesia combines several analgesic methods to optimize pain control while minimizing opioid-related side effects. This approach allows treatment to be tailored to each patient, taking into account their anticipated pain level and history of analgesic use.

5. Post-anaesthetic follow-up

Follow-up after anesthesia is also an essential component in the personalization of anesthesia care. Ongoing assessment of pain levels, side effects and recovery time enables protocols to be adjusted for future procedures.

4. Current practices and future research

Today, several medical institutions are already integrating genetic testing into their preoperative planning process. Clinical studies continue to explore how these tests can be standardized and integrated into routine surgical protocols. The future could see even wider adoption of these practices as sequencing technologies advance and our understanding of gene-environment interactions improves.

Post-operative follow-up and prevention of complications in personalized surgery

Personalized surgery, which relies on the patient's specific characteristics to tailor surgical interventions, requires particular attention to post-operative follow-up and the prevention of complications. This is crucial to ensure not only the immediate success of the operation, but also the long-term health of the patient.

Post-operative follow-up

Post-operative follow-up involves a series of assessments and interventions designed to monitor the patient's recovery from surgery. Studies show that regular follow-up can significantly reduce complication rates. Key elements of follow-up include:

1. **Clinical assessment**: This includes regular visits to assess the patient's general condition, check vital signs, and monitor wound healing.

2. **Pain management**: Adequate pain control is essential for rapid recovery. Individualized protocols can be set up to meet the specific needs of each patient.

3. **Monitoring complications**: Post-operative complications such as infection, bleeding or thromboembolic problems need to be carefully monitored. Tools such as risk scores can help identify high-risk patients.

4. **Rehabilitation**: Physical rehabilitation may be necessary for some patients to restore function and mobility.

5. **Patient education**: Informing patients about warning signs and appropriate home care is fundamental to preventing complications.

Preventing Complications

The prevention of complications in personalized surgery is based on several strategies:

1. **Pre-operative planning**: A thorough pre-operative assessment helps identify individual risk factors (such as comorbidities) that could influence the surgical outcome.

2. **Advanced Surgical Techniques**: The use of less invasive techniques can reduce recovery time and minimize the risk of complications.

3. **Multidisciplinary protocols**: Collaboration between surgeons, anesthetists, nurses and other healthcare professionals is essential to ensure consistent, effective follow-up.

4. **Use of advanced technologies**: The integration of technological tools such as telemedicine enables closer monitoring without the need for frequent physical visits.

5. **Longitudinal follow-up**: Long-term follow-up helps detect any late-onset or recurrent complications at an early stage, enabling prompt intervention.

5. Ethical considerations

Finally, it is important to address the ethical considerations surrounding the use of genetic data in preventive and surgical medicine. Confidentiality of personal data and informed consent are crucial when dealing with sensitive information that could have a significant impact on an individual's medical treatment.

Ethics and informed consent in personalized surgery

Personalized surgery, which refers to the tailoring of surgical interventions to each patient's specific needs, raises complex ethical issues, particularly with regard to informed consent. Informed consent is a fundamental principle of bioethics, which stipulates that patients must be fully informed of the risks, benefits and alternatives of an intervention before giving their consent. In the context of personalized surgery, this notion takes on an even more critical dimension due to the complexity of procedures and the associated uncertainties.

1. Ethics in Personalized Surgery

Fundamental ethical principles include autonomy, beneficence, non-maleficence and justice. Autonomy implies that patients have the right to make decisions about their own bodies after receiving all relevant information. In personalized surgery, where techniques may be innovative or experimental, it is essential that patients understand not only what is being proposed but also why it might be beneficial or risky for them specifically.

2. Informed Consent

The informed consent process must be an ongoing dialogue between doctor and patient. Practitioners must ensure that patients understand the information provided, which may require repeated explanations or the use of visual aids to clarify complex concepts. In addition, it is crucial that consent is obtained without coercion; this means that patients must feel free to ask questions and express their concerns.

3. Practical challenges

In clinical practice, there are several challenges that can impede obtaining adequate informed consent in personalized surgery. These challenges include:

- **Technical complexity**: Customized surgical procedures may involve advanced technologies or innovative approaches that are not well understood by all patients.

- **Uncertainty**: Predictable outcomes may be less clear in individualized treatments, making it difficult for patients to correctly assess risks.
- **Time pressure**: Time constraints in a clinical environment can limit the doctor's ability to provide exhaustive information.

4. Regulatory framework

There is also a regulatory framework that guides the informed consent process in different countries. For example, some legislations require consent to be documented in writing for certain surgical procedures, to ensure legal protection for both patient and practitioner.

Understanding genetic variants in personalized surgery

Personalized surgery, also known as personalized medicine or precision medicine, represents an innovative approach that integrates an individual's genetic information to optimize surgical treatments. This method is based on an understanding of the genetic variants that can influence a patient's response to a specific treatment, including surgical interventions.

1. Understanding genetic variants

Genetic variants are changes in an individual's DNA sequence that can affect various aspects of health, including disease susceptibility, drug response and surgical outcomes. In-depth studies of these variants involve the analysis of nucleotide polymorphisms (SNPs), mutations and other forms of genomic variation. These analyses enable researchers and clinicians to better understand how these differences can influence surgical risk, recovery time and treatment efficacy.

2. Applications in Personalized Surgery

In the context of personalized surgery, genetic information is used to :

- **Patient selection**: Identify those most likely to benefit from a specific surgical intervention.
- **Predicting outcomes**: Assessing how a patient might react to a given procedure based on his or her genetic profile.
- **Adapting surgical techniques**: Modifying surgical approaches based on the patient's genetic characteristics to minimize risk and maximize efficacy.

3. Clinical Studies and Research

Numerous clinical studies have been conducted to explore the impact of genetic variants on various types of surgery, including:

- Oncology surgery, where certain mutations can influence the choice of surgical treatment.
- Orthopedic surgery, where variations in genes linked to bone healing can affect post-operative recovery time.

This research underlines the importance of integrating a DNA-based approach into the surgical decision-making process.

4. Ethical and practical challenges

Despite its potential benefits, the implementation of personalized surgery raises several ethical and practical challenges:

- **Data confidentiality** : The secure management of genetic information is crucial to protecting patient privacy.
- **Unequal access to technologies**: There is a risk that only certain populations will have access to these technological advances, which could exacerbate health inequalities.

5. Future prospects

The future of personalized surgery looks bright with the continuing advance of technologies such as high-throughput sequencing and artificial intelligence. These tools will not only enable a better understanding of genetic variants, but also their integration into standardized surgical protocols.

2. Imaging and personalized modeling

Imaging and personalized modeling in personalized surgery are rapidly expanding fields aimed at improving surgical outcomes through tailored approaches. These techniques rely on the use of advanced imaging data, such as MRI (magnetic resonance imaging), CT (computed tomography) and ultrasound, to create precise three-dimensional models of a patient's anatomical structures. This enables surgeons to plan and simulate surgical procedures with unprecedented precision.

Imaging in Personalized Surgery

Medical imaging plays a crucial role in personalized surgery. Thanks to advanced technologies, doctors can obtain detailed images that reveal not only the morphology of organs, but also their function. For example, MRI can provide information on the vascularization of a tumor, which is essential in determining the best surgical approach. In addition, functional imaging techniques can assess the metabolic activity of specific tissues, providing a more complete picture of the patient's condition.

Imaging Technologies

Medical imaging technologies include computed tomography (CT), magnetic resonance imaging (MRI), ultrasound and nuclear medicine. Each of these modalities offers specific advantages for visualizing anatomical structures and pathologies. For example, MRI is particularly useful for assessing soft tissue, while CT provides excellent bone resolution.

Data analysis

The analysis of data from these imaging modalities is crucial to personalized surgery. Image processing algorithms and artificial intelligence are increasingly used to extract relevant information that can influence the choice of treatment. These tools enable surgeons to better understand patient morphology and identify precise surgical targets.

Integration into the decision-making process

Integrating medical imaging into the surgical decision-making process involves interdisciplinary collaboration between radiologists, surgeons and other healthcare professionals. This not only enables better preoperative planning, but also allows treatment to be tailored to the patient's unique characteristics.

Clinical Applications

The clinical applications of this approach are vast. In the case of cancer, for example, the use of advanced imaging techniques enables tumors to be better targeted while preserving surrounding healthy tissue. Similarly, in the orthopedic field, 3D imaging can help design custom implants adapted to the patient's specific anatomy.

Custom Modeling

Custom modeling refers to the creation of 3D models based on collected imaging data. These models can be used to simulate different surgical strategies even before the patient undergoes surgery. For example, in the case of orthopedic surgery, a 3D model of the patient's skeleton can be used to plan an operation to correct a deformity or implant a prosthesis. This approach not only reduces operating time, but also improves precision and post-operative results.

3D modeling for personalized surgery

3D modeling in personalized surgery represents a significant advance in the medical field, enabling surgeons to plan and execute surgical procedures with greater precision. This approach relies on the use of digital technologies to create three-dimensional models of a patient's anatomical structures from medical images, such as computed tomography (CT) or MRI scans. These models not only enable a better understanding of individual anatomy, but also the simulation of surgical procedures before they are carried out.

1. Creating 3D Models

The first step in 3D modeling is to acquire medical imaging data. Techniques such as computed tomography (CT) and magnetic resonance imaging (MRI) provide detailed images that can be converted into digital models. These images are often processed using specialized software that segments the various anatomical structures, enabling the creation of precise models.

2. Clinical applications

The clinical applications of 3D modeling are vast. In the field of orthopedic surgery, for example, models can be used to design customized implants that fit the patient's anatomy perfectly. Similarly, in neurosurgery, 3D models help to plan complex interventions on the brain by precisely visualizing the relationships between tumors and surrounding brain structures.

3. Benefits

One of the key benefits of this technology is improved surgical outcomes. By enabling surgeons to better understand a patient's unique anatomy, 3D modeling reduces the risk of errors during the operation, and can also reduce the time spent in the operating room. In addition, it facilitates communication between members of the surgical team, and can be used to educate patients about their condition and proposed treatment.

4. Technical challenges

Despite its many advantages, implementing 3D modeling in a clinical setting presents a number of technical challenges. Model accuracy is highly dependent on the quality of the initial imaging data and the software used to generate the model. In addition, there is a growing need for standardization in the methods used so that these technologies can be widely adopted in different medical establishments.

5. Future prospects

As technology continues to evolve, we're likely to see even greater integration of 3D modeling with other emerging technologies such as 3D printing and augmented reality. These innovations could transform not only how surgeries are planned, but also how they are performed, making even greater personalization of surgical care possible.

Clinical Applications

The clinical applications of these technologies are vast. In cardiology, for example, 3D models can help plan complex procedures such as valve repairs or cardiac ablations. In oncology, they enable surgeons to better target tumors while preserving the surrounding healthy tissue. In neurosurgery, these techniques help to navigate critical areas of the brain while minimizing risks.

3. Custom prostheses and 3D printing in surgery.

3D printing, also known as additive manufacturing, has emerged as a revolutionary technology in various fields, including medicine. In particular, its application in personalized surgery has attracted growing interest among researchers and practitioners. This technology makes it possible to create precise anatomical models and customized medical devices that meet patients' specific needs.

3D printing applications in personalized surgery

1. **Anatomical modeling**: One of the most significant applications of 3D printing is the creation of anatomical models based on medical imaging data such as MRI or CT scans. These models enable surgeons to better understand a patient's unique morphology prior to surgery. For example, in the case of complex procedures such as cardiac or orthopedic surgery, these models can help plan the surgical approach and anticipate potential challenges.

2. **Customized implants**: 3D printing also enables the production of customized implants that adapt perfectly to the patient's anatomy. This is particularly relevant in the orthopedic field, where customized prostheses can improve post-operative comfort and functionality. 3D-printed implants can be made from biocompatible materials that promote bone integration.

3. **Surgical tools**: Specific surgical tools can also be created using 3D printing to meet the particular requirements of a given operation. These tools can be designed to optimize precision and reduce operating time, which can have a direct impact on clinical outcomes.

4. **Surgical training**: Another important dimension is the use of 3D-printed models for surgeon training. These models enable students and professionals in training to gain practical experience without risk to real patients.

5. **Personalized treatments**: Beyond direct surgical applications, 3D printing also opens the way to greater personalization of medical treatments. For example, it is possible to print drugs or devices delivering specific therapies tailored to a patient's genetic or physiological profile.

Challenges and ethical considerations

Despite its undeniable advantages, the integration of 3D printing into personalized surgery poses a number of challenges. Regulatory validation of 3D-printed medical devices remains a complex issue, requiring careful attention to ensure their safety and efficacy. In addition, there are ethical concerns regarding the intellectual property linked to the digital designs used to print these devices.

Medical Imaging

Medical imaging encompasses a variety of techniques such as MRI (magnetic resonance imaging), CT (computed tomography), ultrasound and nuclear medicine. Each of these methods provides visual information on the anatomy and physiology of the human body, enabling clinicians to accurately diagnose pathologies.

1. **MRI**: MRI uses powerful magnetic fields and radio waves to generate detailed images of internal organs. It is particularly useful for visualizing soft tissues, such as the brain or muscles.

2. **Computed tomography (CT)**: CT combines several X-ray images to create a cross-sectional view of the body, which is essential for detecting tumors or structural abnormalities.

3. **Ultrasound**: This technique uses sound waves to produce real-time images, often used during pregnancy or to evaluate abdominal organs.

4. **Nuclear medicine**: By using radioactive tracers, this method enables organ function to be assessed, and can help detect certain diseases before they are visible using other imaging methods.

Custom Modeling

Personalized modeling refers to the use of computer models based on individual patient data to simulate various clinical scenarios. This includes:

1. **Anatomical models**: Based on 3D imaging, these models enable doctors to better understand a patient's unique morphology prior to surgery.

2. **Physiological models**: These simulate the normal and pathological functioning of the human body, helping to predict how a patient might respond to a specific treatment.

3. **Computer-aided surgical planning**: thanks to 3D modeling, surgeons can plan their operations with greater precision, reducing the risk of complications.

4. **Targeted therapies**: Modeling also makes it possible to develop personalized treatments based on a patient's specific genetic and biological characteristics.

Clinical Applications

The clinical applications of these technologies are vast:

- **Early diagnosis**: Integrating advanced imaging with modeling enables earlier and more accurate disease detection.

- **Therapeutic monitoring**: clinicians can monitor the evolution of a disease or the effectiveness of a treatment thanks to repeated imaging coupled with model-based analysis.

- **Clinical research**: These tools are also used in clinical trials to evaluate new treatments or medical devices.

Practical work on 3D modernization of pediatric pelvic tumors or malformations

3D modernization of pelvic tumors or malformations in children is a rapidly expanding field that combines digital technology, medical imaging and 3D modeling to improve diagnosis, treatment and surgical planning. This hands-on project aims to familiarize students with the fundamental concepts of this innovative technology, as well as enabling them to apply this knowledge in a clinical context.

Practical work objectives

- **Understanding Basic Concepts**: Students should gain a thorough understanding of pelvic tumors and malformations in children, including their types, causes and clinical implications.

- **Introduction to Medical Imaging**: Familiarize students with the various imaging techniques used to diagnose these conditions, such as ultrasound, computed tomography (CT) and MRI.

- **3D modeling**: Students will learn to use 3D modeling software to create digital representations of tumors or malformations based on imaging data.

- **Clinical applications**: Discuss how these 3D models can be used for surgical planning, patient education and research.

- **Ethics and Clinical Considerations**: Addressing ethical issues related to the use of advanced technologies in the treatment of children.

Practical Activities

- **Case Study**: Analyze several real-life case studies where 3D modeling has been used to treat pelvic tumors in children. Students will be asked to identify the advantages and disadvantages of each approach.

- **Modeling Workshop**: Use specific software (such as Blender or MeshLab) to create a 3D model based on a supplied MRI image of a pelvic deformity. This will include the process of importing medical images, cleaning the data and creating the model.

- **Surgical simulation**: Using the model created, simulate a surgical procedure, discussing the necessary steps and identifying the associated risks.

- **Final presentation**: Each group will present its case study and 3D model to its peers, explaining how it might influence clinical treatment.

- **Ethical discussion**: Organize a discussion on the ethical implications of using 3D models in pediatric treatment, including informed consent and medical confidentiality.

MODULE 3: THERAPEUTIC COMMUNICATION TECHNIQUES

Introduction

Therapeutic communication is an essential area of healthcare, particularly in professions related to psychology, psychiatry and nursing. It refers to the interaction between a healthcare professional and a patient, where the main objective is to establish a relationship of trust that promotes the patient's emotional and psychological well-being. Therapeutic communication techniques are varied and can include active listening, empathy, open questioning, validation of feelings and emotional mirroring.

1. Active listening

Active listening is a fundamental technique that involves not only hearing the words spoken by the patient, but also understanding the underlying meaning. This requires total attention to the patient's verbal and non-verbal language. Active listening helps to create a safe environment where the patient feels understood and respected.

2. Empathy

Empathy is the ability to understand and share another person's feelings. In a therapeutic context, this means that the professional must be able to put themselves in the patient's shoes to better grasp their experiences and emotions. This emotional connection can strengthen the therapeutic relationship and encourage the patient to open up more.

3. Open questioning

Open-ended questioning allows patients to express their thoughts and feelings without being restricted by yes/no answers. This type of questioning encourages a deeper exploration of the patient's problems, facilitating a better understanding of the underlying issues.

4. Validation of feelings

Validating a patient's feelings means recognizing that their emotions are legitimate and worthy of being felt. This can help reduce the stigma associated with emotional or psychological problems, enabling the patient to feel accepted in their experience.

5. Reflecting emotions

Emotional mirroring is a technique in which the professional rephrases what the patient has expressed to show that he or she has understood their feelings. It can also help patients clarify their own thoughts and emotions.

In short, therapeutic communication techniques play a crucial role in establishing an effective relationship between healthcare professional and patient. They not only improve the quality of care provided, but also encourage a deeper healing process by fostering greater mutual understanding.

Chapter 11: Motivational interviewing

Motivational interviewing (MI) is a client-centered approach that aims to strengthen the intrinsic motivation of individuals to change behavior. It was developed in the 1980s by William R. Miller and Stephen Rollnick, primarily to treat addiction problems, but has since been applied to a variety of health fields, including mental health, weight management and medical adherence.

In-depth studies on motivational interviewing

- **Theoretical foundations**: Motivational interviewing is based on several psychological theories, including self-determination theory and the transtheoretical model of change. Self-determination theory emphasizes the importance of intrinsic motivation for lasting change, while the transtheoretical model describes the stages a person goes through when changing a behavior.

- **Key techniques**: Motivational interviewing techniques include active listening, mirroring, summarizing and clarifying personal values. These techniques aim to create an empathetic environment where the customer feels safe to explore ambivalences about change.

- **Clinical applications**: Motivational interviewing has been used successfully in a variety of clinical contexts. For example, studies have shown its effectiveness in the treatment of addictions (alcoholism, smoking), as well as in the management of chronic diseases such as diabetes and hypertension.

- **Training and supervision**: To be effective, practitioners must receive adequate training in motivational interviewing. This includes not only a theoretical understanding of the underlying principles, but also supervised practice to develop the necessary skills.

- **Evaluating effectiveness**: Numerous empirical studies have evaluated the effectiveness of motivational interviewing in comparison with other therapeutic approaches. The results often show that MI can produce significant positive results in terms of commitment to change and improved health outcomes.

Motivational interviewing practices in therapeutic communication

Therapeutic communication is essential in any helping relationship. Motivational interviewing enriches this communication by :

- **Strengthening the therapeutic relationship**: By adopting an empathetic, non-judgmental stance, the practitioner fosters a climate of trust.
- **Exploring ambivalence**: The practitioner helps the client identify his own motivations for change, while acknowledging his hesitations.
- **Goal co-construction**: Instead of imposing external goals, EM encourages customers to define their own goals based on their personal values.
- **Follow-up and adjustment**: Motivational interviewing is not a one-off event; it requires regular follow-up to assess progress and adjust strategies if necessary.

Technique to help patients find their own motivation for change

Motivation to change is a central concept in the field of psychology and behavioral health. Health professionals, including psychologists, counselors and therapists, use a variety of techniques to help their patients discover and strengthen their own intrinsic motivation. This is particularly relevant in the context of cognitive-behavioral therapies (CBT), motivational therapy and other patient-centered approaches.

Techniques to Help Patients Find Their Own Motivation

- **Active Listening** :
- **Definition and principles**: Active listening is based on several fundamental principles, including full attention to the speaker, clarification of messages received, and appropriate feedback. It requires both emotional and cognitive engagement on the part of the healthcare professional.
- **Active listening techniques**: Techniques include :
    - **Paraphrase**: Rephrase what the patient has said to show that you've understood.
    - **Ask open-ended questions**: Encourage patients to express themselves more fully.

    - **Use non-verbal cues**: Maintain eye contact, nod to show you're listening.
    - **Validating emotions**: Acknowledging and validating the patient's feelings to establish an empathic connection.

- **Importance in the medical context**: Active listening is crucial to obtaining accurate information about patient symptoms, understanding their concerns and establishing a collaborative treatment plan. Studies show that when patients feel listened to, they are more likely to follow medical recommendations.

- **Active listening training**: Many communication training programs for healthcare professionals include modules on active listening. These courses can include role-playing, clinical simulations and constructive feedback to improve this skill.

- **Impact on patient satisfaction**: Research indicates that the effective use of active listening can lead to a significant increase in patient satisfaction, a reduction in medical misunderstandings and better adherence to prescribed treatments.

- **Open questions**
  Communication with patients is a fundamental aspect of healthcare, influencing not only patient satisfaction, but also clinical outcomes. Open questions play a crucial role in this dynamic, as they encourage patients to express themselves freely and share relevant information about their state of health.

Importance of Open Questions

Open-ended questions are those that cannot be answered with a simple "yes" or "no". They encourage the patient to expand on their answers, which can provide the healthcare professional with more complete and nuanced information. For example, instead of asking "Are you in pain?", an open-ended question might be "Can you describe how you feel about your pain?". This approach allows the patient to share their personal experience, which can reveal important details about their condition.

Techniques for asking open-ended questions

- **Encourage Expression**: Using phrases like "What's worrying you most at the moment?" or "How is this affecting your daily life?" helps open up discussion.

- **Exploring Feelings**: Asking "How do you feel about your current treatment?" helps to understand the patient's emotional state.

- **Clarifying Information**: A question such as "Can you tell me more about your symptoms?" encourages the patient to provide additional details.

- **Invite to Share the Story**: Phrases like "Tell me how it started" provide a chronological and contextual overview of the disease.

- **Asking for Opinions**: Asking the question "What do you think of your current situation?" gives patients the opportunity to express their thoughts and concerns.

Practical examples

- **On Pain**: Instead of simply asking if the patient is in pain, we could ask: "Can you describe where you feel the pain and how it changes during the day?"

- **Concerning Side Effects**: Rather than asking if the treatment causes side effects, we could say, "What changes have you noticed since you started this treatment?"

- **On Treatment Adherence**: An open-ended question such as "What are your thoughts on the proposed treatment plan?" can help identify potential barriers to adherence.

- **Open questions**: Asking open-ended questions encourages patients to think deeply about their desires and goals. For example, "What motivates you to consider a change now?" opens up a dialogue about their personal motivations.

- **Reflecting feelings**: By reflecting on what the patient is expressing, the therapist can help clarify the underlying emotions driving the desire for change. For example, "It sounds like you're feeling a lot of frustration with your current situation."

- **Positive reinforcement**: Encouraging small victories and celebrating progress can boost patient motivation. Phrases like "You did a great job taking that first step" can be very effective.

4. **Positive reinforcement in therapeutic communication**

Positive reinforcement is an essential technique in therapeutic communication, aimed at encouraging desired behaviors in patients while building their confidence and self-esteem. This approach is based on sound psychological principles and has been extensively studied in clinical psychology and behavior therapy.

Key concepts of positive reinforcement

a) **Definition of positive reinforcement**: Positive reinforcement refers to the addition of a pleasant stimulus after a desired behavior, thereby increasing the likelihood that this behavior will be repeated. In a therapeutic context, this may include verbal praise, encouragement or other forms of recognition.

b) **Importance of trust**: Trust between therapist and patient is crucial to effective treatment. An environment where the patient feels valued and understood fosters better communication and greater openness during sessions.

c) **Communication techniques**: The phrases therapists use to positively reinforce their patients must be carefully chosen. They must be authentic, specific and adapted to the patient's individual context.

Examples of confidence-building phrases

Here are some examples of phrases therapists can use to positively reinforce their patients:

1) **Recognition of efforts** :

   ✓ "I'm really impressed with the effort you've put in this week."

   ✓ "It's great to see how you apply what we've discussed."

2) **Emotion validation** :

- ✓ "It's completely normal to feel this way, and I'm here to support you."
- ✓ "Your feelings are valid, and I thank you for sharing them with me."

3) **Encouragement to continue** :

- ✓ "You're making remarkable progress; keep it up!"
- ✓ "Every little step counts, and I'm proud to see you moving forward."

4) **Capacity building** :

- ✓ "You have the resources within you to overcome these challenges."
- ✓ "Your ability to reflect on your experiences is really impressive."

5) **Creating a safe space** :

- ✓ "This space is a place where you can be yourself without judgment."
- ✓ "I'm here to listen and understand your perspective."

6) **Visualizing Goals**: Helping patients visualize their future after making a change can boost motivation. A phrase like "Imagine how different your life could be if you achieved this goal" can stimulate enthusiasm for change.

5. Visualizing goals in therapeutic communication

Goal visualization in therapeutic communication is a technique that enables practitioners to improve the effectiveness of their interventions. This approach relies on the ability to imagine desired outcomes, which can reinforce motivation and guide actions towards achieving these results. As part of therapeutic communication, visualization can be used to help patients clarify personal goals, overcome emotional obstacles and strengthen their commitment to the therapeutic process.

Key concepts

a) **Definition of visualization**: Visualization is a mental process by which a person creates mental images of desired goals or outcomes. In therapy, this may involve imagining a situation in which the patient has achieved his or her goals or sees himself or herself effectively managing emotions.

b) **Role in therapeutic communication**: Therapeutic communication involves an active exchange between therapist and patient. Visualization helps to establish a deeper connection, enabling the patient to express his or her desires and fears while building self-confidence.

c) **Visualization techniques**: Several techniques can be used, such as :

   a. **Guided visualization**: The therapist guides the patient through an imaginary scenario in which he or she achieves his or her goals.

   b. **Visual diaries**: Encourage patients to draw or write about their goals to create a tangible representation of their aspirations.

   c. **Visual meditation**: using meditation exercises to help patients focus on their goals while reducing anxiety.

d) **Practical examples**:

   a. A patient suffering from social anxiety could be asked to imagine a situation in which he or she successfully interacts with other people, thereby boosting his or her confidence.

   b. A person looking to lose weight could use visualization to imagine themselves reaching their target weight and adopting a healthy lifestyle.

e) **Proven effectiveness**: Studies have shown that visualization can improve not only patient engagement with therapy, but also overall treatment outcomes. The underlying psychological mechanisms include activation of brain areas associated with real-life experiences when imagining future events.

f) **Normalizing Difficulties**: Reassuring the patient that encountering obstacles is normal in any change process can reduce change anxiety. For example, "Many people find it difficult at first, but every little step counts."

g) **Exploring Personal Values**: Discussing the patient's core values can help align his or her goals with what's really important to him or her. A question like "What values do you hold most dear?" can open up an enriching discussion.

6. **Exploring personal values**

a) **Importance of Personal Values**: Personal values influence not only how therapists perceive their clients, but also how they interpret their behavior and emotions. For example, a therapist who values autonomy might encourage clients to make independent decisions, while one who favors collectivization might emphasize interpersonal relationships.

b) **Exploration techniques**: Several techniques can be used to explore personal values in therapy. These include self-reflection exercises in which the therapist examines his or her own values before interacting with the client. Tools such as values questionnaires or open-ended discussions can also help clarify these elements.

c) **Impact on clinical practice**: Awareness of personal values can have a significant impact on clinical practice. For example, a therapist who is aware of his or her biases can better manage his or her emotional reactions to a client's behaviors, thus fostering a more empathetic and less biased approach.

d) **Practical examples**: A concrete example would be a therapist working with a client with different religious beliefs. By exploring his or her own values regarding spirituality, the therapist can avoid imposing his or her own beliefs on the client, while respecting the client's value system.

e) **Training and supervision**: Ongoing training and supervision are essential to help professionals explore their own values. Workshops and discussion groups can provide a safe space to discuss ethical challenges related to value differences between therapist and client.

Best examples

- **Reflection exercise**: Ask therapists to write about their own life experiences that have shaped their values.

- **Role-playing**: Simulate scenarios where value differences might be an issue, so that therapists can practice their response.
- **Constructive Feedback**: Encourage a culture where colleagues can give feedback on how personal values influence their practice.

Examples of Phrases to Seduce Your Patient

1. "I'm here to support you on this journey; what inspires you today?"
2. "Every little step you take is a victory; how can you celebrate that?"
3. "It's normal to have doubts; let's talk about them together."
4. "Imagine yourself six months from now; what would be your greatest accomplishment?"
5. "What resources do you already have inside you that could help you in this process?"

These techniques and phrases aim not only to motivate the patient, but also to establish a solid therapeutic relationship based on trust and empathy.

Chapter 12: Person-centred approach

Introduction

The person-centered approach, developed by Carl Rogers in the 1940s and 1950s, is a method of therapeutic communication that focuses on the client's subjective experience. The approach is based on several fundamental principles designed to create an environment conducive to personal growth and psychological healing.

Fundamental principles of the Person-Centered Approach

1. **Unconditional acceptance**: One of the pillars of this approach is unconditional acceptance, where the therapist offers non-judgmental support to the client. This allows the client to feel free to explore their thoughts and emotions without fear of rejection.

2. **Empathy**: The therapist must demonstrate empathy, i.e. understand and feel what the client is experiencing. This deep understanding helps establish a relationship of trust, essential to the therapeutic process.

3. **Authenticity**: Therapists must be authentic and transparent in their communication. This means sharing one's own feelings and reactions when appropriate, which strengthens the connection between therapist and client.

4. **Customer autonomy**: The person-centered approach values the client's autonomy as an individual capable of making decisions about his or her own life. The therapist's role is to accompany the client on his or her journey, rather than impose solutions.

5. **Subjective experience**: This approach recognizes that each individual has a unique perception of his or her experience. Therapists strive to understand this perspective in order to help clients explore their feelings and thoughts.

Application in Therapeutic Communication

In a therapeutic setting, the person-centered approach promotes open, honest communication between therapist and client. Techniques used include open-ended questions, rephrasing to show that the therapist is actively listening, and validation of the emotions expressed by the client.

This method has been widely adopted in a variety of psychological contexts, including individual therapy, support groups, as well as educational and community settings. It has also influenced other psychotherapeutic approaches by integrating elements such as mindfulness and emotion-based therapies.

In short, the person-centered approach to therapeutic communication provides a powerful framework for fostering a constructive relationship between therapist and client, allowing a safe space for personal exploration and emotional healing.

Techniques based on the next Carl Rogers, emphasizing listening and acceptance

The Carl Rogers approach, also known as person-centered therapy, is based on fundamental principles that emphasize active listening and unconditional acceptance. This method was developed in the 1940s and 1950s by Carl Rogers, a humanist psychologist who revolutionized psychological practice by placing the client at the center of the therapeutic process. The main aim of this approach is to help individuals reach their full potential by fostering an environment in which they feel accepted and understood.

Active Listening

Active listening is an essential skill in Rogers' approach. It involves not only hearing the words spoken by the client, but also understanding the emotional meaning behind them. This requires total attention and empathic presence. Therapists trained in this technique use techniques such as mirroring (rephrasing the feelings expressed by the client) and clarification (asking for clarification in order to better understand) to encourage open communication.

Unconditional Acceptance

Unconditional acceptance is a central concept in person-centered therapy, developed by Carl Rogers. This approach emphasizes the importance of an authentic, empathic therapeutic relationship, in which the therapist accepts the client without judgment. Unconditional acceptance means that the therapist values the client for who they are, regardless of their actions or thoughts. This creates a safe environment that encourages personal growth and emotional exploration.

In-depth studies of acceptance

1. **Concept and importance**: Unconditional acceptance is essential to establishing a relationship of trust between therapist and client. Rogers argued that this acceptance allows the client to feel free to explore their feelings without fear of judgment or rejection. This fosters greater self-understanding and encourages clients to engage in a process of positive change.

2. **Application in therapeutic communication**: In practice, this involves the therapist listening actively and showing empathic understanding of the client's experiences. For example, when a client expresses feelings of shame or guilt, the therapist can respond with affirmations that show understanding of these emotions, while maintaining an attitude of acceptance.

3. **Practical examples**: An effective example might be when the therapist says: "I understand that you feel this way, and it's perfectly normal to have these feelings". This type of response validates the client's emotions while showing him that he's not alone in his experience.

4. **Impact on patients**: Research shows that patients who experience unconditional acceptance are more likely to improve their self-esteem and general well-being. They often feel more motivated to explore their personal problems and work towards solutions.

5. **Clinical results**: Studies have shown that unconditional acceptance contributes not only to client satisfaction with the therapeutic process, but also to positive clinical outcomes, such as a reduction in depressive and anxiety symptoms.

Convincing examples for patients

To convince patients of the effectiveness of unconditional acceptance, it's helpful to use concrete examples:

1. **Testimonials**: Sharing anonymous testimonials from other customers who have benefited from such an approach can help illustrate its effectiveness.

2. **Hypothetical scenarios**: Presenting scenarios in which a patient has overcome his or her obstacles thanks to unconditional acceptance can also be powerful.

3. **Practical demonstrations**: In the first few sessions, the therapist can demonstrate this acceptance by responding to the patient's concerns with empathy and validation.

4. **Education on theory**: Briefly explaining the theory behind the person-centered approach can help patients understand why this method works.

5. **Personalized follow-up**: Offering regular follow-up to discuss the progress made with this approach also reinforces its perceived value to patients.

Practical Techniques

Techniques based on Carl Rogers' approach include :

1. **Reflection**: The therapist rephrases what the client says to show that he or she is actively listening and understands.
2. **Open-ended questions**: These questions encourage customers to express themselves more freely and explore their thoughts and emotions.
3. **Emotional validation**: Acknowledging and validating customers' emotions strengthens their sense of acceptance.
4. **Empathy**: The therapist tries to understand the client's perspective by putting himself in his place.
5. **Gentle confrontation**: When necessary, the therapist can gently address inconsistencies in the client's statements to promote awareness.

Carl Rogers' key techniques in therapeutic communication

1. **Unconditional positive regard**: One of the fundamental techniques of Rogers' approach is the concept of unconditional positive regard. This involves accepting and valuing clients without judgment or conditions. By providing a safe space where clients feel accepted, they are more likely to open up about their thoughts and feelings, leading to deeper self-exploration.

2. **Empathy**: Empathy is another fundamental technique employed by Rogers. It requires therapists to deeply understand and resonate with the client's experiences from their own perspective. This involves active listening, reflecting on what the client has expressed and demonstrating

genuine concern for their feelings. Empathy helps build trust between therapist and client, fostering a stronger therapeutic alliance.

3. **Congruence (Authenticity)**: Congruence refers to the therapist's authenticity in his or her interactions with clients. Rogers believed that therapists should be authentic and transparent about their own feelings, while remaining professional. When therapists demonstrate congruence, this encourages clients to be equally authentic, thus fostering honest dialogue.

4. **Active listening**: Active listening is an essential skill in Rogers' model of therapeutic communication. It involves focusing fully on what the client is saying, rather than passively listening to his or her words. Therapists practice active listening by nodding, maintaining eye contact, summarizing the client's points and asking clarifying questions where necessary.

5. **Reflexive responses**: Reflexive responses involve paraphrasing or summarizing what a client has said to demonstrate understanding and validate feelings. This technique not only shows that the therapist is engaged, but also allows clients to hear their thoughts transcribed back to them, which can lead to new insights.

6. **Facilitating self-exploration**: Rogers emphasized that individuals have an innate capacity for self-understanding and personal growth when given appropriate support. Therapists facilitate this process by asking open-ended questions that encourage clients to explore their thoughts and feelings more deeply.

7. **Non-directive approach**: Unlike other therapeutic modalities that may steer clients toward specific outcomes or solutions, Rogers' person-centered therapy is non-directive. The therapist does not impose his or her views or interpretations, but allows clients to carry on the conversation at their own pace.

Best examples of techniques put into practice

- A therapist practicing unconditional positive respect might say, "I appreciate you sharing this with me; it's okay to feel what you feel."

- To show empathy, a therapist might respond, "I get the impression that you're feeling really overwhelmed right now; I can understand why that might be difficult."
- A congruent response might involve a therapist expressing vulnerability by saying, "I find this topic difficult too; it's normal for both of us to feel uncertain."

Applications of Carl Rogers in therapeutic communication

1. **Client-centered therapy**: At the heart of Rogers' method is the idea that the client is the expert in his or her own experience. Within this framework, the therapist adopts a posture of active listening and empathy to help the client explore his or her feelings and thoughts. For example, in an individual therapy context, a therapist might use techniques such as reformulation and clarification to encourage the client to reflect more deeply on difficult experiences.

2. **Trust and safety**: Rogers stressed the importance of a safe environment where clients can express themselves without judgment. In support groups for people in addiction recovery, for example, creating a space where each participant feels respected and accepted fosters open, honest communication.

3. **Application in education**: Rogerian principles have also been applied in education. Teachers who adopt a student-centered approach encourage autonomy and responsibility in their students. For example, in a classroom where students are encouraged to share their opinions without fear of negative repercussions, there is often an increase in commitment and motivation.

4. **Organizational development**: In the professional context, the concepts developed by Rogers can be used to improve communication within teams. Workshops based on his principles have been implemented to foster a climate of trust between colleagues, leading to improved collaboration and reduced interpersonal conflict.

Practical examples

- **Individual therapy**: A practical example would be a therapist using Rogerian techniques to help a client deal with social anxiety by allowing them to freely explore their fears without judgment.

- **Support groups**: In a self-help group for teenagers with emotional problems, a facilitator trained in Rogersian methods could facilitate open discussions where each participant feels supported.

- **Education**: A teacher who applies these principles might organize sessions where students share their ideas on a given topic, with the assurance that they won't be criticized.

- **Workplace**: When a company implements training based on the Rogersian approach to improve team dynamics, it can lead to a more positive organizational culture.

Chapter 13: Conflict resolution techniques

Managing conflict in a therapeutic setting is an essential skill for mental health professionals. Conflicts can arise for a variety of reasons, including differences of opinion, misunderstandings or unmet expectations between therapist and client. Effective communication is crucial to navigating these delicate situations and fostering an environment conducive to healing.

1. Understanding conflicts

Conflicts in therapy can be classified as intrapersonal (internal conflicts within the client), interpersonal (between client and therapist), or systemic (involving other parties such as the family). Understanding the nature of the conflict is the first step towards resolving it. According to psychological theories, conflicts can often reflect unmet needs or conflicting core values.

2. Communication techniques

Clear, empathetic communication is essential to managing conflict. Techniques include:

- **Active listening**: This involves listening carefully to what the other person is saying without interrupting, while showing empathy.
- **Validating feelings**: Recognizing and validating the customer's emotions can help defuse a conflict situation.
- **Using "I" instead of "you"**: This technique helps prevent the other person from feeling attacked, which can reduce defensiveness.

3. Therapeutic approaches

Different therapeutic approaches offer specific strategies for managing conflicts:

- **Person-centered therapy**: This approach emphasizes unconditional acceptance and empathy, allowing the client to express him/herself freely.
- **Cognitive-behavioural therapy (CBT)**: CBT can help identify and modify dysfunctional thoughts that contribute to conflict.
- **Mediation**: In some cases, involving a neutral third party can help resolve conflicts.

4. Continuing education

Professionals also need to engage in ongoing training to improve their conflict management skills. This can include workshops on intercultural communication, stress management, and other interpersonal skills.

5. Evaluation and reflection

After a conflict, it's crucial to assess what happened and why. Reflecting on one's own reactions, as well as those of the customer, can provide valuable lessons for avoiding similar situations in the future.

In short, managing conflict in a therapeutic setting requires a combination of communication skills, a deep understanding of relationship dynamics, and a willingness to learn continuously.

Chapter14: Empathy and emotional validation

Empathy and emotional validation are fundamental concepts in the field of therapeutic communication. Empathy is defined as the ability to understand and share the feelings of others, while emotional validation is the non-judgmental acknowledgement and acceptance of a person's emotions. Both play a crucial role in establishing an effective therapeutic relationship, fostering an environment where the client feels understood and supported.

Empathy in Communication

Empathy is often considered an essential skill for mental health professionals. It enables the therapist to connect with the client on an emotional level, facilitating a better understanding of the client's experiences. According to Carl Rogers, a pioneer in the field of humanistic psychotherapy, empathy is essential for creating a climate of trust that encourages openness and honesty in the therapeutic relationship (Rogers, 1957). A therapist's ability to feel what his or her client is feeling can also help identify underlying problems that may not be immediately apparent.

Emotional Validation

Emotional validation is a technique that aims to recognize the client's emotions as legitimate and worthy of attention. This approach not only helps to reduce emotional distress, but also boosts the client's self-esteem. By validating emotions, the therapist demonstrates understanding of the client's internal struggles, which can be particularly beneficial for those who have experienced trauma or stressful situations (Linehan, 1993). Validation does not necessarily mean that the therapist approves of the client's behaviours or thoughts; rather, it emphasizes that the emotions felt are understandable given the circumstances.

Interconnection between Empathy and Emotional Validation

Empathy and emotional validation are interconnected; they work together to create a positive dynamic in therapy. An empathic therapist will be more likely to validate the client's emotions, while effective validation often requires an empathic understanding of the feelings being expressed. Together, these skills enable the client to feel heard and respected, which can promote a deeper healing process.

Conclusion

In short, empathy and emotional validation are essential to effective communication in therapeutic settings. They enable clients to explore their emotions safely, while reinforcing their sense of belonging and understanding. Research continues to explore how these skills can be developed in professionals to improve clinical outcomes.

How do you show empathy and validate the patient's emotions

Empathy and emotional validation are crucial elements of therapeutic communication. These skills enable therapists to create a safe and welcoming environment for their patients, fostering greater understanding and emotional support. Here's an in-depth exploration of these concepts.

1. Understanding empathy

Empathy is the ability to understand and share the feelings of others. In the therapeutic context, this involves not only actively listening to the patient, but also recognizing his or her emotions without judgment. Empathy can be divided into two main types:

1. **Cognitive empathy**:

Cognitive empathy, often defined as the ability to understand the emotions and perspectives of others without necessarily feeling those emotions oneself, is a field of study that has attracted growing interest in diverse fields such as psychology, neuroscience and even philosophy. Unlike affective empathy, which involves an emotional response to another's emotional state, cognitive empathy focuses on the cognitive process of understanding the feelings and thoughts of others.

In-depth studies on cognitive empathy

- **Definition and distinction**: Cognitive empathy is often distinguished from affective empathy. According to research, it involves cognitive mechanisms that enable individuals to decode emotional signals and make inferences about what others might be thinking or feeling. This can be particularly useful in complex social contexts where navigating interpersonal dynamics is crucial.
- **Neuroscience of empathy**: Neuroscience studies have identified certain brain regions associated with cognitive empathy, notably the prefrontal cortex and the superior temporal cortex. These areas are involved in social

processing and theory of mind, which is the ability to attribute mental states to oneself and others.

- **Practical applications**: Cognitive empathy plays an essential role in various fields, such as medicine, where it can improve communication between doctors and patients, or in education, where it can foster better understanding between teachers and students. For example, a teacher who can identify a pupil's emotional difficulties can adapt his or her teaching approach to better meet individual needs.
- **Concrete examples**: A practical example of cognitive empathy could be seen in a situation where a manager has to assess the morale of his team. By understanding the underlying concerns expressed by his employees during a meeting, he can adjust his managerial strategies to create a more positive environment.
- **Personal development**: Cognitive empathy can also be cultivated through a variety of techniques, such as emotional intelligence training or perspective-taking exercises that take into account different points of view in difficult discussions.

Dimensions of Empathy

- **Cognitive Dimension**: This refers to the ability to understand the emotions and perspectives of others. In a therapeutic setting, this implies that the therapist is able to grasp what the patient is feeling without necessarily experiencing these emotions themselves.

- **Affective dimension**: This dimension concerns the ability to feel what the other is feeling. An empathic therapist can not only understand the patient's pain or joy, but also experience an appropriate emotional response.

Empathy Practices in Therapeutic Communication

Empathetic practices can include:

- **Active listening**: This involves listening carefully to what the patient is saying, while showing non-verbal signs of attention (such as nodding or maintaining eye contact). Active listening helps create a safe space for the patient to express himself freely.

- **Emotional Validation**: Acknowledging and validating the patient's emotions is essential. For example, saying "I understand how difficult this must be for you" can help the patient feel heard and understood.

- **Reflection**: Rephrase what the patient has said to show that you have understood his or her feelings. For example, "It sounds like you're feeling very frustrated by this situation."

Application examples

a) **Cognitive Behavioral Therapy (CBT)**: In a CBT session, a therapist might use empathic techniques to help a patient suffering from social anxiety. By listening carefully and validating the patient's fears about social interactions, the therapist can establish an alliance that facilitates the exploration of these fears.

b) **Person-centered therapy**: Carl Rogers developed this approach, which relies heavily on empathy. An example would be a therapist who uses empathic reflections to encourage a client to explore his or her deepest feelings without judgment.

c) **Crisis intervention**: When an individual is going through an intense emotional crisis, such as after a tragic loss, a professional trained in empathy can offer support by actively listening and providing a comforting presence.

d) **Support groups**: In contexts such as chronic illness support groups, empathy between members fosters an environment where everyone feels free to express their personal struggles.

e) **Family therapy**: In family therapy, each member may need to be heard and understood by the others; here, empathy plays a key role in resolving family conflicts.

2. **Emotional empathy** :

Affective empathy, often defined as the ability to feel and understand the emotions of others, plays a crucial role in therapeutic communication. It enables therapists to establish an authentic connection with their clients, fostering an environment conducive to openness and healing. In this in-depth analysis, we'll examine the theoretical foundations of affective empathy, its practical applications in therapeutic contexts, and illustrative examples.

Theoretical Foundations of Affective Empathy

Affective empathy is often distinguished from cognitive empathy. Whereas cognitive empathy involves intellectual understanding of others' emotions, affective empathy focuses on emotional sharing. Theorists such as Carl Rogers have emphasized the importance of empathy in client-centered therapy. Rogers argued that for a client to feel understood and accepted, the therapist must demonstrate genuine empathy.

Practical Applications in Therapeutic Communication

- **Active listening**: Active listening is an essential skill that accompanies affective empathy. It involves not only hearing the client's words, but also perceiving the underlying emotions. For example, a therapist might say, "I sense that you are very sad about what has happened", showing that he or she recognizes and validates the client's feelings.

- **Emotional Validation**: Emotional validation is another key application of affective empathy. By acknowledging and validating the client's feelings, the therapist helps create a safe space where the client can explore their emotions without judgment. For example, a therapist might say, "It's perfectly normal to feel overwhelmed in this situation," which helps the client feel understood.

- **Emotional Reflection**: Emotional reflection involves rephrasing or paraphrasing what the client has expressed, while focusing on their feelings. This can help customers clarify their thoughts and emotions. For example: "You seem really frustrated by this situation", allows the customer to explore their frustration further.

- **Use of Non-Verbal Language**: Body language also plays an essential role in empathic communication. Appropriate eye contact, open posture and responsive facial expressions can reinforce the customer's sense of empathy.

- **Creating a Therapeutic Alliance**: Affective empathy helps to establish a solid therapeutic alliance between therapist and client. A good alliance is often correlated with positive results in therapy.

Illustrative examples

- **Example 1**: A patient suffering from social anxiety might share his fears about an upcoming social interaction. A therapist using affective empathy might respond, "I can imagine how difficult this must be for you; many people feel this way in social situations." This response shows the patient that they are not alone in their experience.

- **Example 2**: When a client talks about a recent loss, an empathic therapist might say, "Losing someone you love is incredibly painful; it's normal for you to feel that pain." This validates the client's feelings while strengthening their emotional bond.

- **2. Importance of emotion validation**

Emotional validation is essential because it helps patients feel understood and accepted. It can reduce their sense of isolation and enable them to explore their feelings more deeply without fear of being judged.

3. Impact on the therapeutic relationship

Good empathy and effective validation of emotions can build trust between therapist and patient, facilitating a space where the patient feels free to express their thoughts and feelings without reservation.

4. Further training

Professionals need to engage in ongoing training to improve their empathy and emotional validation skills. Workshops, seminars and specialized training courses can help develop these essential skills.

5. In-depth conclusion to the therapeutic communication study

Therapeutic communication is a fundamental aspect of healthcare, playing a crucial role in the healing process and patient well-being. It encompasses a series of interactions between the healthcare professional and the patient, aimed at establishing a relationship of trust, encouraging the expression of emotions and facilitating the understanding of medical information. This study highlighted several key elements that underline the importance of effective communication in the therapeutic setting.

First and foremost, it is essential to recognize that therapeutic communication is not limited to the transmission of medical information. It also involves active listening, where the professional fully engages with the patient's concerns. Active listening not only gathers relevant information about the patient's condition, but also validates his or her feelings and experiences. This helps to create a climate of psychological safety, where the patient feels free to express his or her fears and needs.

Secondly, non-verbal communication plays just as important a role as spoken words. Gestures, facial expressions and tone of voice can convey powerful messages that complement or contradict words. Therefore, adequate training for healthcare professionals in the non-verbal aspects of communication is crucial to improving the effectiveness of interactions with patients.

Furthermore, it is imperative that professionals adopt a patient-centered approach. This means that every interaction must be tailored to the patient's individual needs, taking into account their cultural, social and emotional context. Such an approach not only promotes adherence to treatment, but also improves the patient's overall satisfaction with the care received.

Finally, this study also highlights the importance of ongoing communication training for healthcare professionals. Communication skills can be developed and honed over time through workshops, simulations and other educational methods. Better communication preparation can reduce misunderstandings and significantly improve clinical outcomes.

In conclusion, therapeutic communication is an indispensable element in medical care. By integrating effective active listening practices, paying attention to non-verbal communication, adopting a patient-centered approach and investing in ongoing professional training, we can significantly improve the patient experience and overall health.

Chapter 15: Confidentiality and respect for patients

Introduction

Confidentiality and respect for patient rights are fundamental elements in the healthcare field. These concepts are essential not only to protect patients' personal information, but also to maintain trust between patients and healthcare professionals. Confidentiality implies that all information concerning a patient, including his or her state of health, medical history and personal preferences, must be kept secret and may not be disclosed without the patient's explicit consent. This is particularly relevant in a context where digital technologies facilitate information sharing, but also increase the risk of data breaches.

Respect for patients' rights encompasses several aspects, including the right to information, the right to informed consent and the right to dignity. Patients need to be informed about their medical conditions and proposed treatments, so that they can make informed decisions about their health. Informed consent is crucial; it ensures that patients fully understand the implications of treatments before they consent to them. What's more, every patient has the right to respectful treatment that takes into account their human dignity.

Issues relating to patient confidentiality and rights are also reinforced by various pieces of legislation such as HIPAA (Health Insurance Portability and Accountability Act) in the United States or the General Data Protection Regulation (GDPR) in Europe. These laws aim to protect personal data and ensure that individuals' rights are respected in all aspects of healthcare.

In conclusion, the importance of confidentiality and respect for patient rights cannot be underestimated. They constitute not only an ethical obligation for healthcare professionals, but also a fundamental right for every individual receiving medical care. Protecting these principles is essential to promote a healthy relationship between patients and healthcare providers, and to ensure ethical medical practice.

Importance of confidentiality Respect for patients Respect for patients' rights.

Confidentiality and respect for patient rights are fundamental to the healthcare industry. Not only are these principles essential to establishing a relationship of trust between healthcare professionals and patients, they are also anchored in laws and regulations that protect patients' personal information.

The importance of confidentiality

1. **Patient-practitioner trust**:

Trust between patient and practitioner is a fundamental element of healthcare. It influences not only patient satisfaction, but also clinical outcomes. The relationship of trust is based on several factors, including communication, empathy, the practitioner's perceived competence, and respect for the patient's values and preferences.

1. The importance of trust in the therapeutic relationship

Trust is often described as central to the therapeutic relationship. Patients who trust their doctors are more likely to follow medical recommendations, share relevant information about their condition and express their concerns. Studies show that this trust can reduce patient anxiety and improve engagement in the care process (Hall et al., 2002).

2. Factors influencing confidence

Several factors influence the level of trust a patient places in a practitioner:

- **Professional competence**: Patients often assess a doctor's competence by his or her qualifications, experience and ability to clearly explain diagnoses and treatments.

- **Communication**: Open, honest communication is crucial to building trust. Practitioners who actively listen to their patients and answer their questions foster a climate of security.

- **Empathy**: Empathy plays a key role in establishing an emotional connection between practitioner and patient. Practitioners who demonstrate a sincere understanding of patients' concerns reinforce their sense of security.

3. Consequences of low confidence

Low confidence can have adverse consequences for the patient's health. It can lead to non-adherence to prescribed treatments, a reluctance to seek medical care, or even a deterioration in general health (Mechanic & Meyer, 2000). It can also lead to mistrust of the healthcare system in general.

4. Confidence-building strategies

To build trust in the patient-practitioner relationship, several strategies can be implemented:

- **Ongoing training**: Healthcare professionals need to engage in ongoing training to keep abreast of best practices in communication and interaction with patients.
- **Patient feedback**: Encouraging feedback enables practitioners to adjust their approach according to patients' specific needs.
- **Patient-centered practices**: Adopting a patient-centered approach that respects the patient's personal values helps build a strong bond based on trust.

2. Legal protection:

Numerous laws, such as the HIPAA (Health Insurance Portability and Accountability Act) in the USA, impose strict standards on the protection of medical information. Failure to comply with these laws can result in severe penalties for healthcare establishments.

1. Privacy

Confidentiality is an essential pillar of therapeutic communication. It implies that all information shared by the patient must be protected from unauthorized disclosure. Personal data protection laws, such as the General Data Protection Regulation (GDPR) in Europe, impose strict obligations on healthcare professionals regarding the handling and storage of sensitive information.

2. Informed Consent

Informed consent is another crucial element in therapeutic communication. This means that patients must be fully informed of proposed treatments, including potential risks and benefits, before agreeing to any medical intervention. This process must be carefully documented to avoid any ambiguity or misunderstanding that could lead to litigation.

3. Legal responsibilities

Healthcare professionals have a legal responsibility to their patients, which includes the obligation to act with diligence and competence. In the event of negligence or breach of established ethical standards, they may face prosecution. Ongoing training in medical law is therefore essential to ensure that practitioners keep abreast of legislative and regulatory developments.

4. Ethical practices

Ethical practices in therapeutic communication are also fundamental to establishing a relationship of trust between patient and healthcare professional. These include empathy, active listening and respect for the patient's point of view. These elements contribute not only to improving the patient experience, but also to reducing the legal risks associated with poor communication.

5. Vocational training

Finally, it is imperative that professionals are trained not only in clinical techniques, but also in the legal and ethical aspects of their practice. Educational programs integrating these dimensions can help prepare future practitioners to navigate the complexities of therapeutic communication while respecting legal requirements.

3. Professional ethics:

Professional codes of ethics, such as those established by the American Medical Association (AMA) or France's Code de déontologie médicale, stress the importance of respecting patient privacy as a moral duty.

Professional ethics in therapeutic communication is a crucial field of study that examines the moral and ethical principles that guide interactions between mental health professionals and their clients. This discipline focuses on several aspects, including confidentiality, informed consent, patient autonomy and cultural competence.

1. Privacy

Confidentiality is a fundamental pillar of therapeutic communication. Professionals must ensure that all information shared by the client remains private, except in situations where there is an imminent risk to the safety of the client or others. Violation of this trust can have serious consequences for the client's well-being and damage the therapeutic relationship.

2. Informed Consent

Informed consent is another essential aspect of ethical therapeutic communication. This implies that the professional must provide the client with all the necessary information concerning the proposed treatment, including its potential risks and benefits, so that the client can make an informed decision about his or her participation.

3. Patient autonomy

Respecting patients' autonomy means recognizing their right to make decisions about their own lives and treatment. Practitioners must encourage clients to express their preferences and actively participate in the decision-making process.

4. Cultural competence

Cultural competence is also crucial to ethical therapeutic communication. Professionals need to be aware of cultural differences that may influence the client's perception of treatment, and adapt their approach accordingly to respect these diversities.

5. Ethical practices

Ethical practices in therapeutic communication also include ongoing training for professionals so that they can keep abreast of best practices and developments in the field of medical ethics.

4. Psychological impact:

Therapeutic communication is an essential area of study in psychology and psychotherapy, as it plays a crucial role in the patient's healing process. The psychological impact of this communication can be analyzed across several dimensions, including the relationship between therapist and patient, the communication techniques used, and the effects on the patient's mental well-being.

1. The therapeutic relationship

The quality of the relationship between therapist and patient is often regarded as one of the most decisive factors in effective treatment. According to Carl Rogers, a pioneer of client-centered therapy, an authentic, empathetic and non-judgmental relationship fosters an environment conducive to healing. Studies show that when patients feel understood and accepted, they are more likely to open up their emotions and engage fully in the therapeutic process.

2. Communication techniques

The specific techniques used by therapists can also influence the psychological impact on patients. For example, active listening - which involves not only hearing the words spoken, but also understanding the underlying feelings - is essential to establishing a meaningful connection. Approaches such as reformulation or emotional mirroring enable patients to better understand their own emotional experiences.

3. Effects on mental well-being

Research indicates that positive interactions in the therapeutic context can lead to a reduction in depressive and anxiety symptoms in patients. In addition, good communication can boost self-esteem and foster a sense of autonomy in individuals undergoing therapy. Longitudinal studies have shown that those who benefit from effective communication with their therapist often report lasting improvements in their mental health.

4. Communication barriers

It's also important to explore the barriers that can hinder effective communication in the therapeutic environment. Factors such as patient anxiety, cultural or linguistic biases, and differences in communication styles can create misunderstandings or diminish treatment effectiveness.

5. Recommended practices

To maximize the positive psychological impact of communication in therapy, practitioners are advised to adopt a client-centered approach that values empathy, transparency and collaboration. Ongoing training in interpersonal skills and awareness of patients' diverse cultural needs are also essential to enhancing this dynamic.

5. **Informed Consent**:

Informed consent is a fundamental principle in health and therapeutic care. It is a process by which a patient is informed of the risks, benefits and alternatives to a treatment or intervention, enabling him or her to make an informed decision about his or her health. This concept rests on several pillars: patient autonomy, transparency of the information provided by the healthcare professional, and the patient's ability to understand this information.

1. Basic principles of informed consent

Informed consent is based on respect for individual autonomy. According to Beauchamp and Childress (2013), it is essential for patients to be fully informed in order to exercise their right to decide what happens to them. This involves not only a clear explanation of medical procedures, but also an assessment of the patient's understanding.

2. Therapeutic communication

Therapeutic communication plays a crucial role in the informed consent process. Healthcare professionals need to adopt an empathetic approach that is adapted to patients' individual needs. According to McCabe (2004), good communication fosters not only understanding but also trust between patient and practitioner, which is essential to obtaining truly informed consent.

3. Barriers to informed consent

There are several barriers to informed consent, including cultural differences, varying levels of education and cognitive biases that can influence a patient's perception of the information received (Fisher & Mendez, 2016). Professionals need to be aware of these factors in order to adapt their communication.

4. Best practices

To ensure effective informed consent, several practices can be implemented:

- Use of visual tools to explain treatments.
- Regular checks on patient comprehension.
- Encouragement to ask questions (Kirkpatrick & Kirkpatrick, 2015).

5. Ethics and legislation

The ethical framework surrounding informed consent is also supported by laws in many countries that protect patients' rights (Beauchamp & Childress, 2013). These laws stipulate that consent must be obtained prior to any medical intervention.

Respecting patients' rights

1. Right to information:

In-depth, practical studies of patient information law focus on the legal and ethical obligations of healthcare professionals regarding the communication of information to patients. This area of law is essential to ensure that patients are fully informed about their condition, available treatments, associated risks and possible alternatives. This is part of the broader framework of respect for patient autonomy and the right to make informed decisions about their own health.

1. The legal framework

The patient's right to information is often governed by national and international laws designed to protect patients' rights. For example, in France, the Public Health Code stipulates that all patients have the right to be informed about their state of health, which includes the right to access their medical records. Similarly, the European Convention on Human Rights underlines the importance of informed consent in the medical context.

2. Medical ethics

Medical ethics play a crucial role in the patient's right to information. Ethical principles such as respect for autonomy, beneficence and non-maleficence oblige healthcare professionals to provide clear, comprehensible information. This implies not only effective verbal communication, but also appropriate documentation.

3. Clinical practices

In clinical practice, it is essential that doctors adopt a patient-centered approach when conveying information. This means adapting their communication to the patient's level of understanding, using simple language and regularly checking that the patient has understood the information provided.

4. Legal implications

Failure to respect the right to information can lead to legal consequences for healthcare professionals, including legal action for malpractice or negligence. Courts often consider whether a patient has been properly informed before agreeing to treatment or surgery.

5. Technological innovations

With the advent of digital technologies, there are also new challenges when it comes to patient information. Electronic medical records (EMRs) offer easier access to medical information, but also raise questions about the confidentiality and security of personal data.

2. Autonomy:

Patient autonomy and respect for patient rights are fundamental concepts in medical ethics and health law. Autonomy refers to an individual's capacity to make informed decisions about his or her own health and treatment, while respect for patient rights implies recognition and protection of those decisions. These principles are at the heart of modern medical practice, and are supported by various legal and ethical frameworks.

In-depth studies on patient autonomy

- **Definition of autonomy**: Autonomy is often defined as the right of an individual to make choices about his or her own life, including medical decisions. This implies not only the cognitive ability to understand relevant information, but also the freedom to choose without coercion.

- **Legal framework**: In many countries, the right to autonomy is protected by laws that guarantee patients the right to be informed about their state of health, the treatments available and the associated risks. Informed consent laws require healthcare professionals to provide patients with all the information they need to make informed decisions.

- **Medical ethics**: Ethical principles such as respect for autonomy, beneficence (acting in the patient's best interest), non-maleficence (doing no harm) and justice play a crucial role in clinical practice. Respect for autonomy requires clear communication between doctor and patient, fostering an environment where patients feel free to express their preferences.

- **Clinical practices**: Implementing respect for patient rights in clinical practices includes the use of tools such as advance directives, which enable patients to express their wishes regarding future care if they are unable to communicate these wishes themselves.

- **Contemporary challenges**: Despite the recognized importance of autonomy, several challenges persist in its effective implementation. These include inequalities in access to information, cultural differences in the perception of autonomy, and situations where the patient's decision-making capacity may be compromised.

3. **Access to medical records**:

The right of access to medical records is a fundamental aspect of patients' rights, often governed by specific laws and regulations in various countries. This right enables patients to consult their medical information, understand their state of health, and actively participate in decisions concerning their treatment.

Legal and ethical framework

The legal framework surrounding access to medical records varies from country to country, but is generally based on fundamental ethical principles such as respect for human dignity, confidentiality and informed consent. In many countries, data privacy laws, such as the General Data Protection Regulation (GDPR) in Europe or the Health Insurance Portability and Accountability Act (HIPAA) in the US, set strict standards for accessing and sharing medical information.

Importance of Informed Consent

Informed consent is a key principle that must be respected when accessing medical records. Patients must be informed of their rights and understand how their data will be used. This also means that healthcare professionals must ensure that patients understand the implications of sharing their medical information with other parties.

Best Practices for Access to Medical Records

Healthcare facilities need to put in place clear procedures to facilitate access to medical records, while guaranteeing the security and confidentiality of information. This may include:

1. **Staff training**: Make medical staff aware of patients' rights and the appropriate procedures for accessing records.

2. **Secure IT systems**: Use secure electronic systems that protect data from unauthorized access while allowing easy access for patients.

3. **Transparency**: Provide clear information on how to request access to your own medical records.

4. **Recourse mechanisms**: Establish channels through which patients can contest a refusal of access or report a potential violation of their rights.

5. **Ongoing assessment**: Implement a regular assessment of medical record access practices to identify and correct any shortcomings in terms of patient rights.

4. Protection against discrimination:

Protecting patients' rights is a crucial area of healthcare, aimed at ensuring that all individuals receive fair treatment, free from discrimination based on race, gender, age, sexual orientation, socio-economic status or any other personal characteristic. In-depth studies on this subject highlight the different forms of discrimination that can occur in healthcare systems, and propose practices to protect patients' rights.

1. Legal and ethical framework

Laws and regulations play a vital role in protecting patients' rights. In many countries, there is specific legislation prohibiting discrimination in healthcare. For example, the Civil Rights Act in the United States prohibits racial discrimination in various fields, including healthcare. In addition, ethical principles such as respect for patient autonomy and justice are fundamental to ensuring fair practice.

2. Training and awareness-raising

Ongoing training of medical staff is essential to reduce unconscious prejudice and promote a culture of inclusiveness. Educational programs can help raise awareness of discrimination issues and provide healthcare professionals with the tools to treat all patients with dignity and respect.

3. Corporate policies

Hospitals and other healthcare establishments must establish clear policies regarding non-discrimination. This includes the development of protocols for reporting and dealing with cases of discrimination, as well as a commitment to regular monitoring of these practices to ensure their effectiveness.

4. Community involvement

Involving communities in the development and evaluation of healthcare services can also help reduce discrimination. Feedback from patients from diverse backgrounds helps to adapt services to the specific needs of each group.

5. Continuous search

Research plays a key role in identifying equity gaps in healthcare. Quantitative and qualitative studies can reveal how different groups are affected by discrimination within the medical system, enabling decision-makers to develop targeted interventions.

5. Remedies for Violations:

Patients' rights are a set of ethical and legal principles that guarantee the respect, dignity and autonomy of individuals in the context of healthcare. These rights include, among others, the right to information, the right to confidentiality, the right to informed consent and the right to fair treatment. However, despite these protections, violations can occur. It is therefore crucial to explore the in-depth studies and redress practices available to patients in the event of such violations.

1. Legal framework for patients' rights

The legal framework surrounding patients' rights varies from country to country, but is generally based on a number of international and national instruments. For example, the Universal Declaration of Human Rights (1948) and the International Covenant on Economic, Social and Cultural Rights (1966) establish fundamental standards regarding health as a human right. In addition, each country has its own laws protecting patients' rights. In France, for example, Law no. 2002-303 of March 4, 2002 on patients' rights and the quality of the healthcare system was a major turning point in the formal recognition of patients' rights.

2. Types of violation

Violations can take many forms:

- **Violation of informed consent**: Patients must be informed about their condition and the proposed treatments, so that they can freely give their consent.
- **Breach of confidentiality**: Unauthorized disclosure of medical information is a serious violation.
- **Discrimination in access to care**: Inequalities based on ethnic origin, socio-economic status or other factors are also considered a violation.

3. Recourse mechanisms

Redress mechanisms for violations of patients' rights may include:

- **Complaints to regulatory bodies**: In many countries, there are governmental or independent agencies where patients can lodge complaints.
- **Legal action**: Victims may also choose to take legal action against healthcare providers or medical establishments.
- **Mediation**: Some institutions offer a mediation process to resolve disputes without resorting to formal legal proceedings.

4. Role of non-governmental organizations (NGOs)

NGOs play a crucial role in protecting and promoting patients' rights. They raise public awareness of potential violations and often provide legal support to victims. Organizations such as Médecins Sans Frontières and Amnesty International work actively to defend human rights in the medical field.

5. Empirical studies

Empirical research has been carried out to assess the actual impact of violations on patients' mental and physical health, as well as on their trust in the healthcare system. These studies often show that when rights are not respected, this can lead to a significant deterioration in the patient's general well-being.

Conclusion

The study of confidentiality and respect for patient rights is of crucial importance in the healthcare field. Confidentiality refers to the protection of an individual's personal and medical information, while respect for patient rights encompasses a set of ethical and legal principles that ensure patients are treated with dignity, respect and autonomy.

Confidentiality is essential to establishing a relationship of trust between patient and healthcare professional. When patients know that their information will be protected, they are more inclined to share sensitive details about their health, enabling professionals to provide appropriate and effective care. Moreover, breaches of confidentiality can have serious consequences, both psychologically and legally.

Respect for patients' rights also includes the right to information, the right to informed consent, and the right to privacy. These rights are often framed by national and international laws designed to protect individuals against potential abuses in the healthcare system. For example, the Declaration of Helsinki and laws such as HIPAA (Health Insurance Portability and Accountability Act) in the USA set clear standards for the protection of personal data.

In conclusion, it is imperative that healthcare establishments implement robust policies to guarantee confidentiality and respect patients' rights. This requires ongoing training for healthcare professionals in medical ethics, as well as in current data protection laws. Raising public awareness of their healthcare rights is also essential to promote an environment where every individual feels safe and respected in their interactions with the medical system.

Appendix 1: Practical work

Practical work is an essential pillar of medical training. It transforms theoretical knowledge into applicable skills, ensuring that future doctors are optimally prepared for the demands of their profession. Here are the main reasons why they are essential:

1. **Reinforcing theoretical learning**
   Practical work enables students to put into practice the concepts learned in theory classes. This fosters an in-depth understanding of biological, anatomical, physiological and pathological mechanisms.

2. **Developing practical skills**
   Medicine is a discipline based on practical skills. Practical work offers the opportunity to handle instruments, perform specific techniques (e.g. blood sampling, satures) and become familiar with diagnostic and therapeutic protocols.

3. **Improved clinical decision-making**
   In a controlled environment, students learn to analyze clinical cases and make diagnoses, reinforcing their ability to make decisions in real-life situations.

4. **Developing precision and dexterity**
   Practical work enables you to acquire the precise gestures needed for medical practice, whether for surgical procedures or delicate manipulations.

5. **Simulation of clinical experiments**
   Practical work, sometimes combined with realistic simulations, helps students prepare for the clinical situations they will encounter with real patients.

6. **Ethics and communication training**
   Working on practical cases, students learn to interact with simulated or real patients, developing their listening skills, empathy and respect for ethical standards.

7. **Encouraging critical thinking and research**
   Practical work provides opportunities for observation, analysis and critical reasoning. They also encourage students to ask questions and take part in research projects.

8. **Preparing for working life**
   Through practical work, students acquire skills that are directly transferable to their professional practice. This reduces their anxiety and potential errors when entering the medical world.

1. Practical work on Regeneration of Damaged Tissue with Bone Marrow Cells

Introduction

Regeneration of damaged tissue is a crucial area of research in regenerative medicine. Bone marrow cells, notably hematopoietic stem cells and mesenchymal stem cells, play a fundamental role in this process. The aim of this practical work is to explore the mechanisms by which these cells can contribute to the repair and regeneration of damaged tissue.

Practical work objectives

- **Understanding the role of stem cells**: Students will study the different types of cells present in bone marrow and their regenerative potential.
- **Analyze regeneration mechanisms**: It will be essential to explore how these cells interact with the tissue environment to promote healing.
- **Evaluate clinical applications**: Students will need to examine how this knowledge is applied in the treatment of injuries and degenerative diseases.

Methodology

- **Literature review**: Students will begin with an in-depth review of scientific articles and books dealing with tissue regeneration and the role of stem cells.
- **In vitro experimentation**: If possible, students will set up a cell culture using bone marrow-derived stem cells to observe their behavior in response to various stimuli.
- **Clinical case studies**: Analysis of case studies where the use of stem cells has led to a significant improvement in tissue regeneration.

Discussion

The results obtained will enable the students to assess the potential efficacy of stem cell-based therapies for treating a variety of conditions, such as heart injuries, bone injuries and neurodegenerative diseases.

2. Practical work: Complete and detailed presentation of Phytoscience Cellular Biotherapy

Introduction to Phytoscience Cellular Biotherapy

Cellular biotherapy is a therapeutic approach that uses living cells to treat various diseases. In the context of phytoscience, this method relies on the use of medicinal plants and plant extracts to promote health and well-being. An integral part of traditional medicine in many cultures, phytotherapy has seen its effectiveness enhanced by advances in biotechnology and cell biology.

1. Theoretical foundations of Cellular Biotherapy: Cellular biotherapy is based on several fundamental principles:

- **Stem cells**: Stem cells are undifferentiated cells capable of transforming into different cell types. They play a crucial role in tissue regeneration and can be used to treat degenerative diseases.

- **Phytomedicines**: Plant extracts contain a multitude of bioactive compounds (such as flavonoids, alkaloids and terpenes) that can modulate immune responses and promote healing.

- **Synergy between plants and cells**: the interaction between stem cells and phytotherapeutic extracts can enhance the efficacy of treatments, promoting the repair of damaged or diseased tissue.

2. Clinical applications: Phytoscience cell biotherapy has applications in a variety of fields:

- **Oncology**: Using plant extracts to boost the immunity of cancer patients, while reducing the side effects of conventional treatments such as chemotherapy.

- **Autoimmune diseases**: Stem cell therapies can help restore immune balance in patients suffering from autoimmune diseases.
- **Tissue regeneration**: Plant extracts can be used to stimulate tissue regeneration after injury or surgery.

3. Study methodology: To carry out this practical work, students are advised to adopt a rigorous methodological approach:

- **Bibliographic research**: Identify and analyze relevant clinical studies on the combined use of stem cells and phytotherapeutic extracts.
- **Case studies**: Present concrete examples where this biotherapy has been successfully applied.
- **Critical analysis**: Evaluate the potential advantages, disadvantages and ethical challenges associated with these treatments.

4. Future prospects: Current research is paving the way for several promising prospects:

- **Personalized treatment**: With advances in genetic technologies, it will be possible to tailor therapies to each patient's specific needs.
- **Integration into the conventional medical system**: Growing recognition of the effectiveness of alternative medicine could lead to its wider integration into the conventional medical system.
- **Sustainable development**: Focusing on the sustainable use of plant resources could also help preserve biodiversity while improving access to healthcare.

3. Practical work on Robotic Pediatric Surgery

Introduction to Pediatric Robotic Surgery

Pediatric robotic surgery is an innovative branch of medicine that uses robotic systems to perform surgery on pediatric patients. This approach improves precision, reduces surgical trauma and speeds up recovery in young patients.

Surgical robots, such as the da Vinci system, are designed to give surgeons greater visualization and control during delicate procedures.

Practical work objectives

- **Understanding the Fundamentals of Robotic Surgery**: Students should become familiar with the basic principles of robotic surgery, including the technologies used and how they work.
- **Analyze Advantages and Disadvantages**: A critical assessment of the advantages (such as faster recovery and less pain) versus the disadvantages (such as high cost and the need for specialized training) must be carried out.
- **Study Clinical Cases**: Students will be asked to review several case studies where robotic pediatric surgery has been used, analyzing clinical outcomes and impact on patient care.
- **Hands-on simulations**: Using surgical simulators to practice specific robotic techniques, enabling students to gain practical experience in a controlled environment.
- **Discussion Ethics**: Address ethical considerations related to the use of robotic technology in pediatrics, including implications for informed consent and equitable access to care.

Methodology

- **Bibliographical research**: Students should consult academic articles, specialized books and medical journals to deepen their knowledge of the subject.
- **Group work**: Organize group discussions to share findings and debate different perspectives on the use of robotic surgery in pediatrics.
- **Final presentation**: Each group will present its findings in the form of an oral presentation or scientific poster at a seminar dedicated to pediatric surgery.

4. Practical work on the development of a surgical technique: Foetoscopy

Fetoscopy is a surgical technique used to examine the fetus in utero and, in some cases, to treat pathological conditions. The procedure is performed using an endoscope inserted into the uterus via the abdominal or vaginal route. The aim of this practical work is to enable students to understand the fundamental principles of fetoscopy, its historical development, its clinical indications, as well as the techniques and ethical considerations surrounding it.

Practical work objectives

- **Understanding the Anatomical and Physiological Basics** :
    - Study the anatomy of the fetus and uterus.
    - Analyze the physiological implications of fetoscopy for the fetus and mother.
- **History and development of fetoscopy** :
    - Look for early attempts at fetoscopy.
    - Identify the technological advances that have led to the development of this technique.
- **Clinical indications** :
    - Discuss pathological conditions that may require fetoscopy (e.g. congenital malformations, fetal anemia).
    - Examine the eligibility criteria for this procedure.
- **Surgical techniques** :
    - Describe the steps involved in the fetoscopic procedure.
    - Study the instruments used during the procedure.
- **Ethical considerations and associated risks** :
    - Analyze potential risks for mother and fetus.

- Discuss the ethical implications of in utero surgery.

Methodology

- **Bibliographic research**: Students will need to consult academic articles, specialized books on obstetrics and gynecology, and medical journals to deepen their understanding of the subject.
- **Case study**: Students will be able to analyze real-life case studies where fetoscopy has been used successfully or has led to complications.
- **Practical simulation**: If possible, organize a laboratory simulation using anatomical models to practice handling surgical instruments in a fetoscopic context.

Conclusion

This practical work aims to provide students with a thorough understanding not only of the technical aspects of fetoscopy, but also of its clinical and ethical implications. By integrating theory and practice, they will be better prepared to tackle this complex surgical technique in their future medical careers.

5. Practical work on Endoscopic and Genetic Screening for Colorectal Cancer

Colorectal cancer is one of the most common types of cancer worldwide, and early detection is crucial to improving survival rates. Screening methods mainly include endoscopic screening and genetic testing. This practical work aims to familiarize students with these two approaches, focusing on their importance, techniques, and clinical implications.

1. Introduction to Colorectal Cancer

Colorectal cancer develops in the colon or rectum, and may be asymptomatic in its early stages. Early detection through screening methods is essential to reduce the mortality associated with this disease.

2. Endoscopic screening

Endoscopic screening includes procedures such as colonoscopy, which visually examines the inside of the colon and rectum. This method not only detects polyps or early lesions, but also allows biopsies to be taken or polyps to be removed during the procedure.

- **Technique**: Colonoscopy uses a flexible tube equipped with a camera to visualize the intestinal mucosa.
- **Preparation**: Patients must follow a specific diet before the examination to ensure good visibility.
- **Advantages**: Direct detection of early lesions, possibility of immediate intervention.
- **Disadvantages**: Risks associated with the procedure (perforation, bleeding), patient discomfort.

3. Genetic screening: Genetic screening is used to identify individuals at high risk of developing colorectal cancer due to hereditary factors.

- **Genetic tests**: tests such as those identifying mutations in the APC or MLH1 genes can predict increased susceptibility to colorectal cancer.
- **Genetic counseling**: Patients with a significant family history may benefit from genetic counseling before undergoing testing.
- **Ethical implications**: Genetic screening raises ethical issues concerning confidentiality and potential discrimination in relation to results.

4. Comparison of endoscopic and genetic screening: Both methods have their advantages and disadvantages:

Criteria	**Endoscopic screening**	**Genetic Screening**
Sensitivity	High	Varies according to the genes tested

Invasiveness	Invasive	Non-invasive
Cost	High	Variable
Preparation required	Yes	No

5. Conclusion

The choice between endoscopic and genetic screening will depend on the patient's individual profile, including age, family history and personal preferences. An integrated approach combining these two methods may offer a better screening strategy for reducing the incidence of colorectal cancer.

6. Practical work on Laparoscopic training in Urology

Introduction to Laparoscopy in Urology

Laparoscopy is a minimally invasive surgical technique that has revolutionized the field of urology. It enables surgeons to perform complex procedures with smaller incisions, thereby reducing recovery time and post-operative complications. In learning this technique, it is essential that students acquire not only technical skills, but also a thorough understanding of the underlying anatomical and physiological principles.

Practical work objectives

- **Theoretical understanding :**
    - Study the fundamental principles of laparoscopy.
    - Analyze the indications and contraindications of laparoscopic procedures in urology.

- **Technical skills :**
    - Master the use of laparoscopic instruments.
    - Develop skills in suturing and tissue manipulation.
- **Practical Simulation :**
    - Participate in simulation sessions using anatomical models or virtual simulators.
    - Observe and participate in real surgical procedures under supervision.
- **Evaluation and Reflection :**
    - Evaluate individual performance in simulations.
    - Write a reflective report on the learning experience, including challenges encountered and lessons learned.
- **Methodology**

- **Theoretical sessions:** Lectures will be given to introduce the key concepts of laparoscopy in urology.
- **Practical workshops:** Students will work in small groups to practice on mannequins or simulators.
- **Clinical observation:** Students will have the opportunity to observe laparoscopic surgeries performed by experienced urologists.
- **Constructive feedback:** After each practical session, feedback will be given to help improve technical skills.

Conclusion

Learning laparoscopy in urology requires an integrated approach combining theory, practice and critical reflection. This practical work aims to prepare students to become proficient in this advanced surgical technique, essential in the modern field of urology.

7. Practical work: echo-endoscopic evaluation and treatment of adenocarcinoma

Echo-endoscopic evaluation and management of adenocarcinoma of the middle rectum are crucial topics in gastroenterology and oncology. Echo-endoscopy, or endoscopic ultrasound (EE), is an imaging technique that combines endoscopy and ultrasound to provide detailed images of the layers of the rectal wall and surrounding structures. This method is particularly useful in the evaluation of rectal tumors, as it can determine the depth of tumor invasion and identify regional lymph nodes.

Echo-Endoscopy evaluation

- **Principles of Echo-Endoscopy**: Echo-endoscopy uses an ultrasound probe inserted into the rectum to obtain images in real time. The sound waves emitted by the probe reflect off the tissues, enabling visualization of the different layers of the rectal wall (mucosa, submucosa, muscularis and serosa).

- **Indications**: EE is indicated to assess the depth of tumor invasion (T stage) and to detect lymph node metastases (N stage). It is often used when other imaging methods such as computed tomography (CT) or magnetic resonance imaging (MRI) do not provide sufficient information.

- **Interpretation of results**: The results of echo-endoscopy must be interpreted with care. Adenocarcinoma of the middle rectum can be classified according to the TNM system (Tumor, Node, Metastasis). The depth of invasion (T) is determined by the extension of the tumor into the layers of the rectum.

Treatment of Middle Rectal Adenocarcinoma

- **Staging**: Following echo-endoscopic evaluation, it is essential to staging the cancer in order to determine the appropriate treatment. Staging includes not only local assessment, but also complementary imaging to look for distant metastases.

- **Therapeutic options** :
    - **Surgery**: Surgical resection remains the main treatment for early stages.
    - **Chemotherapy and radiotherapy**: For more advanced or inoperable stages, neoadjuvant chemotherapy or radiotherapy may be considered prior to surgery.
    - **Post-operative follow-up**: Regular follow-up with endoscopic monitoring and imaging is essential to detect any early recurrence.
- **Multidisciplinarity**: Management must involve a multidisciplinary team including gastroenterologists, medical oncologists, surgeons and radiologists, to optimize the patient's therapeutic pathway.

8. Practical Work on Laser Treatment of Couperose

Introduction

Couperose, also known as telangiectasia, is a skin condition characterized by the appearance of small, dilated blood vessels, often visible on the face. It can be caused by a variety of factors, including genetics, sun exposure, hormonal changes and environmental conditions. Laser treatment has become a popular method for reducing the appearance of couperose by targeting the abnormal blood vessels without damaging the surrounding skin.

Practical work objectives

- **Understanding the pathophysiology of rosacea**: Students need to research and explain how blood vessels dilate and become visible.
- **Study the different types of lasers used**: Students should examine the types of lasers (such as the pulsed dye laser and the Nd:YAG laser) and their mechanism of action.
- **Analyze treatment indications and contraindications**: It's essential that students identify who can benefit from laser treatment and who should avoid it.
- **Assess potential side effects**: Students should discuss possible side effects of laser treatment, such as hyperpigmentation or skin irritation.

- **Case studies**: Using fictitious case studies, students will propose a suitable treatment plan for a patient with couperose.

Methodology

- **Literature search**: Students should consult academic articles, specialized books and medical journals to gather relevant information on every aspect of laser treatment.
- **Critical analysis**: They will have to assess the quality of the sources used and discuss the results obtained in their research.
- **Oral presentation**: At the end of the practical work, each student or group of students will present their findings to the class.

Conclusion

Laser treatment of rosacea represents a significant advance in the field of dermatology. This practical work will enable students to acquire a thorough understanding not only of therapeutic techniques, but also of the ethical and practical considerations associated with these procedures.

9. Laser photocoagulation of retinal vessels

Laser photocoagulation of retinal vessels is an essential procedure in the treatment of various ocular pathologies, including diabetic retinopathy, retinal vein occlusions and neovascularization. This technique uses a laser beam to coagulate retinal tissue, which can help stabilize or improve vision by reducing retinal edema and preventing disease progression.

Indications for laser photocoagulation

- **Diabetic retinopathy**: Photocoagulation is often indicated to treat proliferative forms of diabetic retinopathy. The main aim is to reduce the risk of vision loss by destroying the abnormal neovessels that form on the retina.

- **Retinal vein occlusion**: In the case of central or branchial vein occlusion, photocoagulation can be used to treat associated macular edema, helping to improve visual acuity.

- **Choroidal neovascularization**: Patients with age-related macular degeneration (AMD) can benefit from photocoagulation to destroy the abnormal blood vessels that cause subretinal leakage and hemorrhage.

- **Intravitreal hemorrhages**: Photocoagulation may also be indicated in certain cases of intravitreal hemorrhages caused by neovessels, to prevent further complications.

- **Preventing post-surgical complications**: After certain surgical procedures on the retina, such as vitrectomy, preventive photocoagulation can be performed to minimize the risk of secondary neovascularization.

Technical considerations

- **Type of laser used**: Argon lasers are commonly used because of their ability to coagulate effectively without damaging surrounding tissue.

- **Patient selection**: Careful evaluation must be carried out prior to the procedure to ensure that the patient meets the indication criteria and that the potential benefits outweigh the associated risks.

- **Post-procedural follow-up**: Regular follow-up is essential after photocoagulation to monitor the patient's progress and detect any complications.

10. Practical Work: Overview of Surgical Techniques and Development of Medical Devices

Introduction

Surgery and drug device development are two interconnected fields that play a crucial role in modern medicine. This hands-on work aims to explore the techniques used in these two disciplines, focusing on recent innovations, traditional methods, and the impact of technology on clinical outcomes.

I. Surgical techniques

Minimally invasive surgery

Laparoscopic surgery is a technique that uses small incisions and specialized instruments to perform operations with less tissue trauma. This method shortens recovery time and reduces the risk of infection.

Advances in robotics, such as the da Vinci system, enable surgeons to perform complex procedures with greater precision.

Traditional Surgery

Despite the rise of minimally invasive techniques, open surgery remains essential for certain procedures requiring direct exposure of internal organs.

The fundamental principles of surgical hygiene and general anesthesia continue to be crucial to patient safety.

Advanced Techniques

The use of intra-operative imaging (such as MRI or CT scan) enables surgeons to visualize anatomical structures in real time, improving the precision of interventions.

Computer-aided surgical navigation is also booming, offering precise guidance during delicate operations.

II. Development of Medical Devices

Drug Delivery Devices

Targeted delivery systems, such as nanoparticles and liposomes, enable precise administration of drugs directly to diseased cells while minimizing systemic side effects.

Implantable devices, such as insulin pumps or pacemakers, offer continuous management of chronic diseases.

Emerging Technologies

3D printing is used to create customized medical devices tailored to the patient's specific needs.

Biosensors integrated into medical devices enable real-time monitoring of a patient's physiological parameters.

Regulations and Ethics

The development of new medical devices is subject to strict regulations to guarantee their safety and efficacy before they are put on the market.

Ethical considerations surrounding animal and human experimentation are essential to the research and development process.

Conclusion

An overview of the techniques used in surgery and the development of medical devices reveals a dynamic field where technological innovation is continually transforming medical practice. It is essential that students understand not only these techniques, but also their clinical and ethical implications.

11. Practical Work on Digital Stimulation Applied to Surgery and the Development of Medical Devices

Introduction

Digital stimulation has become an essential tool in the field of surgery and medical device development. It encompasses a variety of technologies, including 3D modeling, augmented reality (AR), and computer simulations, which enable surgeons to plan and execute procedures with greater precision. In addition, these technologies facilitate the development of new medical devices by enabling virtual testing prior to their physical manufacture.

Practical work objectives

- **Understanding the basic principles of digital stimulation**: Students will need to familiarize themselves with the fundamental concepts associated with digital simulation, including the software used for modeling and analysis.

- **Exploring surgical applications**: Students will examine how these technologies are applied in various types of surgery, including orthopedic, cardiovascular and neurological.

- **Analyzing the development of medical devices**: Particular attention will be paid to how digital stimulation contributes to innovation in the development of medical devices such as implants, prostheses and drug delivery systems.

- **Assess the impact on clinical outcomes**: Students will be asked to research case studies demonstrating the effectiveness of digital techniques in improving surgical outcomes and therapeutic development.

- **Developing a practical project**: Working in groups, students will create a project using simulation software to design an innovative surgical procedure or medical device.

Methodology

- **Bibliographical research**: Students will use academic resources to deepen their knowledge of the subject.
- **Hands-on workshops**: Practical sessions will be organized to enable students to use software specific to surgical simulation.
- **Presentations**: Each group will present its project to its peers to encourage the exchange of ideas and constructive criticism.

Conclusion

This practical work aims to provide students with an in-depth understanding of the growing importance of digital stimulation in the medical field. By combining theory and practice, they will be better prepared to integrate these technologies into their future professional careers.

12. Practical work on esophageal motor disorders

Introduction

Esophageal motor disorders are conditions that affect the ability of the esophagus to transport food from the mouth to the stomach. These disorders can manifest as symptoms such as chest pain, difficulty swallowing (dysphagia), regurgitation and gastro-oesophageal reflux. This practical work aims to deepen understanding of these disorders, their etiology, diagnosis and treatment options.

Practical work objectives

- **Understanding Types of Esophageal Motor Disorders**: Students will identify and describe the different types of esophageal motor disorders, including:
  - Achalasia
  - Esophageal spasms
  - Lower esophageal sphincter dysfunction
- **Analyze Clinical Symptoms and Signs**: Students will examine how these disorders manifest themselves clinically and what the associated symptoms are.
- **Exploring Diagnostic Methods**: Students will become familiar with diagnostic techniques used to evaluate esophageal motor disorders, such as:
  - Esophageal manometry
  - Endoscopy
  - X-ray with barium
- **Evaluate Treatment Options**: An analysis of different therapeutic approaches will be required, including:
  - Medications (e.g. proton pump inhibitors)
  - Endoscopic procedures
  - Surgery (such as myotomy for achalasia)
- **Study the Psychological Impact**: Students will also need to consider the psychological impact these disorders can have on patients' quality of life.

Methodology

Students will be divided into groups to conduct in-depth research on a specific type of esophageal motor disorder. Each group will be asked to prepare a presentation that includes:

- A presentation on the chosen disorder.
- A discussion of diagnosis and treatment.
- A case study illustrating a fictitious patient with this disorder.

Conclusion

This practical work will enable students to acquire in-depth knowledge of esophageal motor disorders, while developing their research and presentation skills.

13. Practical work: Management of benign esophageal strictures

Introduction

Benign esophageal strictures are non-cancerous narrowings that can lead to difficulty swallowing (dysphagia), chest pain and other complications. Management of these strictures requires a multidisciplinary approach, involving both medical interventions and patient management strategies. This practical work aims to provide students with a thorough understanding of the methods of diagnosis, treatment and follow-up of benign esophageal strictures.

Practical work objectives

- Understand the causes and types of benign stenosis.
- Explore the diagnostic methods used to identify esophageal strictures.
- Discuss available treatment options, including endoscopic dilatation, surgery and medical treatments.
- Assess the importance of post-treatment follow-up and long-term management.

Methodology

- **Bibliographic research:** Students should consult academic books, scientific articles and specialized journals on the subject to acquire a solid theoretical base.

- **Case Study:** Students will be divided into groups and each group will be given a fictitious clinical case of a patient with benign esophageal stenosis. They will be asked to analyze the case and propose an appropriate diagnostic and therapeutic plan.

- **Practical simulation:** use of anatomical models or virtual simulations to practice the endoscopic techniques used in esophageal dilatation.

- **Class discussion:** Each group will present its findings to the rest of the class, followed by a guided discussion of the different approaches and their clinical justifications.

- **Final evaluation:** Writing of a detailed report on the case studied, including a critical review of the therapeutic options chosen and their clinical relevance.

Conclusion

The management of benign esophageal strictures is a complex field requiring a thorough understanding of both theory and practice. This practical work will enable students to acquire the skills needed to approach this clinical problem with confidence.

14. Practical work on the Drug Treatment of Gastric Acidity

Introduction

Gastric acidity, often caused by disorders such as gastro-oesophageal reflux disease (GERD), gastric ulcers and gastritis, is a common health problem requiring an appropriate therapeutic approach. This practical work aims to explore the different drug treatments available to manage gastric acidity, focusing on their mechanism of action, indications, side effects and clinical considerations.

Practical work objectives

- **Understanding the Mechanisms of Gastric Acidity**: Students will examine how gastric acid is produced in the stomach, and what factors may contribute to excessive production.

- **Explore drug classes**:
    - **Antacids**: Understanding their role in neutralizing gastric acid.
    - **Proton Pump Inhibitors (PPIs)**: Investigating their mechanism of action and efficacy in the treatment of acid-related diseases.
    - **H2-receptor antagonists**: Analyze how these drugs reduce acid secretion.
    - **Mucosal protectors**: Evaluate their use in protecting the gastric mucosa.
- **Evaluate side effects**: Students will be asked to identify and discuss the side effects associated with each class of medication.
- **Clinical Case Studies**: Students will be invited to examine case studies where different treatments have been applied, discussing results and possible alternatives.
- **Discussion of Non-Medicinal Approaches**: While this work focuses on drug treatment, it is essential to also address lifestyle modifications that can help manage gastric acidity.

Methodology

Students will have to carry out in-depth research using academic books, scientific articles and medical encyclopedias to gather relevant information. They will then write a detailed report presenting their findings, accompanied by a critical analysis of the treatments studied.

Conclusion

This practical work will enable students to deepen their understanding of the drug treatment of gastric acidity, while developing their research and critical analysis skills.

15. Practical Work on the Clinic of Chronic Inflammatory Bowel Diseases

Introduction

Chronic inflammatory bowel disease (IBD), comprising mainly Crohn's disease and ulcerative colitis, represents a complex group of pathologies characterized by chronic inflammation of the gastrointestinal tract. This practical work aims to deepen clinical understanding of IBD, focusing on its etiology, pathophysiology, clinical manifestations, as well as diagnostic and therapeutic approaches.

Practical work objectives

- **Understanding the etiology of IBD**: Exploring the genetic, environmental and immunological factors that contribute to the development of IBD.
- **Analyze pathophysiology**: study mechanisms of inflammation and immune responses associated with IBD.
- **Identify clinical manifestations**: Recognize typical and atypical symptoms of IBD patients.
- **Review diagnostic methods**: Discuss the tools used to diagnose IBD, including endoscopy, imaging and laboratory tests.
- **Evaluate treatment options**: Analyze available treatments, including anti-inflammatory drugs, immunosuppressants and biological therapies.

Methodology: Students will be divided into groups to explore different aspects of IBD. Each group will :

- Conduct a literature review on the assigned topic.
- Prepare an oral presentation or scientific poster.
- Participate in a class discussion about their findings.

Detailed content

- **Etiology**
    - Studies show that genetic predisposition plays a crucial role in the development of IBD. Mutations in genes such as NOD2 have been identified as risk factors.
    - Environmental factors include diet, smoking and exposure to certain infectious agents.

- **Pathophysiology**
    - An inappropriate immune response lies at the heart of IBD pathophysiology. Excessive activation of T lymphocytes and increased production of pro-inflammatory cytokines are observed in these patients.
    - Intestinal dysbiosis (imbalance of the microbiota) has also been implicated in triggering and aggravating inflammation.
- **Clinical manifestations**
    - Common symptoms include chronic diarrhea, abdominal pain, weight loss and fatigue.
    - Complications such as intestinal fistulas or colorectal cancer may also occur in some patients.
- **Diagnostic methods**
    - Endoscopy with biopsy is considered the gold standard for diagnosing IBD.
    - Imaging tests such as MRI or CT scans can be used to assess the extent of the disease.
- **Therapeutic options**
    - Treatments include non-steroidal anti-inflammatory drugs (NSAIDs), corticosteroids, immunomodulators and biological therapies specifically targeting certain inflammatory pathways.
    - Surgery may be necessary in certain advanced or complicated cases.

Conclusion

This practical work will enable students to acquire an in-depth understanding of chronic inflammatory bowel disease, both theoretically and practically. They will be encouraged to develop a critical approach to the various diagnostic and therapeutic approaches available.

16. Practical work on infusion therapy for ulcerative colitis

Introduction

Ulcerative colitis is a chronic inflammatory bowel disease that mainly affects the colon and rectum. It is characterized by episodes of bloody diarrhea, abdominal pain and general fatigue. Management of this disease can include a variety of treatments, including infusion therapy, which involves administering drugs directly into the circulatory system via a vein. This practical work aims to explore the various facets of this therapeutic approach.

Practical work objectives

- **Understanding ulcerative colitis**: Study the causes, symptoms and complications associated with this disease.
- **Explore treatment options**: Analyze the different treatments available for ulcerative colitis, with an emphasis on infusion therapy.
- **Evaluate the efficacy of infusions**: Review clinical studies and results concerning the use of infusions in the treatment of ulcerative colitis.
- **Discuss side effects**: Identify potential side effects associated with infusion therapy.
- **Develop a care plan**: Develop a care plan incorporating infusion therapy for a fictitious patient with ulcerative colitis.

Methodology

- **Literature search**: Students should consult academic articles, specialized books and medical journals to gather relevant information on ulcerative colitis and its treatment.
- **Case studies**: Analyze real-life case studies where infusion therapy has been used to treat patients with ulcerative colitis.
- **Group discussion**: Organize a class discussion on the advantages and disadvantages of infusion therapy compared with other forms of treatment.

- **Report content:** The final report should include :
    - An introduction to ulcerative colitis.

- A section detailing the mechanisms of action of drugs administered by infusion (such as anti-TNF or immunosuppressive agents).
- A critical analysis of relevant clinical studies.
- A summary table of possible side effects.
- A personalized care plan based on a fictitious clinical scenario.

17. Practical work on the diagnosis and treatment of facial lesions of the spleen

Introduction

Facial lesions of the spleen, although less common than other types of lesions, require special attention because of their potential impact on the patient's overall health. This practical work aims to familiarize students with the diagnostic methods and treatment options available for these lesions.

Practical work objectives

- **Understanding Facial Lesions**: Students should be able to identify the different types of facial lesions that can affect the spleen, including trauma, infection and neoplasia.

- **Diagnostic techniques**: Students will learn to use various diagnostic techniques such as clinical examination, medical imaging (such as ultrasound and CT scans), and possibly biopsies to establish an accurate diagnosis.

- **Therapeutic approaches**: Treatment of facial lesions of the spleen may include surgical intervention, medical treatment or active surveillance. Students will need to explore these different options.

- **Clinical cases**: Students will work on simulated clinical cases to apply their theoretical knowledge to practical situations.

Methodology

- **Bibliographic research**: Students will begin by conducting bibliographic research on the subject, using medical encyclopedias, specialized books and academic articles.

- **Case Analysis**: Each student will receive a fictitious clinical case describing a patient with a facial lesion associated with spleen. They will be asked to analyze the case, make a diagnosis and propose a treatment plan.

- **Oral presentation**: At the end of the practical work, each student will present his or her findings to his or her peers, encouraging the exchange of ideas and the development of communication skills.

- **Assessment :** Students will be assessed on their ability to :
  - Correctly identify lesion types.
  - Effective use of diagnostic tools.
  - Propose an appropriate treatment plan.
  - Clearly communicate their results during oral presentations.

Conclusion

This practical work will enable students to gain a thorough understanding of the diagnosis and treatment of spleen-related facial lesions. By combining theory and practice, they will be better prepared to deal with these situations in their future medical careers.

18. Practical work on adrenal tumor surgery

Introduction

Adrenal tumor surgery is a specialized field of medicine that requires a thorough understanding of the anatomy, physiology and pathologies associated with the adrenal glands. Adrenal tumors can be benign or malignant and include adenomas, carcinomas and pheochromocytomas. This practical course aims to provide students with hands-on experience in the evaluation, diagnosis and surgical treatment of adrenal tumors.

Practical work objectives

- **Anatomical understanding**: Students should acquire a detailed knowledge of the anatomy of the adrenal glands, including their vascularization and innervation.
- **Clinical Assessment**: Students will learn to recognize symptoms associated with adrenal tumors, such as hypertension, metabolic disorders and endocrine manifestations.
- **Surgical techniques**: Familiarize students with the different surgical approaches to adrenal tumor removal, including laparoscopy and open surgery.
- **Histopathological analysis**: Introduction to the histopathological analysis of surgical specimens to determine the benign or malignant nature of the tumor.
- **Post-operative management**: Understand the post-operative care required for patients who have undergone surgery for an adrenal tumor, including hormonal monitoring and oncological follow-up.

Practical Activities

- **Anatomy sessions**: Use of anatomical models or medical images to study the position and structure of the adrenal glands.
- **Case studies**: Analysis of real clinical cases where students will have to diagnose the type of adrenal tumor based on the symptoms presented by the patient.
- **Surgical simulation**: Participation in a surgical simulation where students can practice operating techniques on a simulated model before observing a real operation.
- **Visit to a Surgical Department**: Organization of a visit to a hospital department where adrenal tumor surgery is performed, in order to observe the surgical process at first hand.

- **Ethical discussion**: Debate on the ethical considerations surrounding the surgical treatment of adrenal tumors, particularly with regard to informed consent and choice of treatment.

Conclusion

This practical work will enable students not only to acquire theoretical knowledge, but also to apply this knowledge in a practical setting, reinforcing their preparation to become competent professionals in the field of endocrine surgery.

19. Practical work on testicular torsion surgery

Testicular torsion is a surgical emergency requiring rapid intervention to save the affected testicle. This practical work aims to familiarize students with the clinical, diagnostic and surgical aspects of this condition.

Practical work objectives

- **Understanding Pathology**: Students need to understand what testicular torsion is, its causes, symptoms and consequences if not treated promptly.

- **Clinical Diagnosis**: Students will learn to recognize the clinical signs of testicular torsion, including acute pain in the scrotum, swelling and nausea.

- **Surgical techniques**: Particular attention will be paid to the surgical techniques used to treat testicular torsion, including scrotal exploration and testicular fixation (orchidopexy).

- **Post-operative management**: Students will also need to familiarize themselves with the post-operative care required to ensure optimal patient recovery.

Practical work content

1. Case Study: Students will be divided into groups and each group will be given a fictitious clinical case of a patient with symptoms of testicular torsion. They will have to:

- Analyze the patient's medical history.
- Identify clinical signs.
- Propose a diagnostic plan including physical examinations and imaging tests (such as Doppler ultrasound).

2. Surgical simulation: Use of anatomical models or simulators to practice :

- Scrotal incision.
- Exploring internal structures.
- Torsion detection and treatment.
- Testicular fixation by orchidopexy.

3. Discussion Ethics: Students will discuss the ethical implications of caring for a minor patient with testicular torsion, including informed consent and communication with parents.

4. Final presentation: Each group will present its conclusions on the clinical case studied, and on the surgical techniques used during the simulation.

Conclusion

This practical work will enable students to gain a thorough understanding of testicular torsion, both theoretically and practically, while developing essential clinical skills.

20. Practical work on valve disease

Introduction to Valvulopathy

Valvulopathies are conditions that affect the heart valves, which are essential to the proper functioning of the heart. They fall into two main categories: stenosis (narrowing of the valves) and insufficiency (leakage of the valves). Valvulopathies can have a variety of causes, from congenital malformations to degenerative diseases and infections such as endocarditis.

Pedagogical Objectives

- Understand the anatomy and physiology of the heart, with particular emphasis on the role of the valves.

- Identify the different types of valvulopathy and their etiologies.
- Analyze the clinical symptoms associated with valvulopathy.
- Explore diagnostic methods, including echocardiography and other imaging techniques.
- Discuss treatment options, including medication, reconstructive surgery or valve replacement.

Practical Activities

- **Clinical Case Study:** Students will receive a clinical file detailing a patient with a specific valvulopathy (e.g. aortic stenosis). They will be asked to analyze the symptoms, make a differential diagnosis and propose a treatment plan.

- **Echocardiographic simulation**: use of echocardiography software to visualize different valvulopathies. The students will be asked to identify the abnormalities present on the echocardiographic images and discuss their clinical significance.

- **Bibliographic research:** Students will be asked to research a specific valve disease (e.g. mitral insufficiency) in medical journals and encyclopedias to understand its impact on public health.

- **Oral presentation:** Each student or group of students will prepare an oral presentation on a chosen valve disease, including its causes, symptoms, diagnosis and available treatments.

- **Ethical discussion:** Organize a debate on the ethical implications of surgical versus medical treatment of valvulopathy in different age groups.

21. Practical Work on Obesity and its Impact on Fertility

Introduction: Obesity is a major public health problem with significant implications for various aspects of health, including fertility. This practical work aims to explore the links between obesity and fertility, examining underlying physiological mechanisms, reproductive consequences and intervention strategies.

Practical work objectives :

- Understand the definitions and classifications of obesity.
- Analyze how obesity affects fertility in men and women.
- Study the biological mechanisms by which obesity influences reproduction.
- Evaluate possible interventions to improve fertility in obese individuals.

Suggested activities :

- **Literature search:** Students are expected to conduct in-depth research on the subject of obesity and fertility using reliable academic sources. They should focus on recent studies that examine the link between these two topics.

- **Report Writing:** Each student will be required to write a detailed report of approximately 2000 words that addresses:

    - Definition of obesity (BMI, classifications).
    - The effects of obesity on the endocrine and reproductive systems.
    - Gender differences in the impact of obesity on fertility.
    - Results of relevant clinical studies.

- **Case Study:** Students will analyze a case study of an individual or group who has experienced fertility problems related to obesity. They will discuss contributing factors and potential solutions.

- **Oral presentation:** At the end of the practical work, each student will present their findings to their peers, highlighting the key points discovered during their research.

- **Group discussion:** Organize a class discussion where each student shares his or her thoughts on the subject, enabling an exchange of ideas and a better collective understanding of the issues surrounding obesity and fertility.

Conclusion: This practical work will enable students not only to acquire theoretical knowledge on the subject but also to apply this knowledge in a practical context, thus reinforcing their understanding of the complex implications of obesity on reproductive health.

22. Practical work: The operation to remove diseased testicles

Operation to remove diseased testicles, known as orchiectomy, is a surgical procedure that may be required in several medical contexts. The procedure is often performed in cases of testicular cancer, severe infection or trauma. As part of a practical assignment for students, it would be relevant to explore various aspects of this operation, including medical indication, surgical technique, potential complications and ethical considerations.

Practical work objectives

- **Understanding medical indications**: Students should research and discuss the reasons why an orchiectomy might be recommended. This includes exploring types of testicular cancer (such as seminoma and non-seminoma), as well as non-cancerous conditions that may require this procedure.

- **Surgical technique**: Students should examine the procedure itself, including pre-operative steps (such as anesthesia and patient preparation), operative technique (incision, testicular removal) and necessary post-operative care.

- **Potential complications**: A thorough analysis of the risks associated with orchiectomy is essential. This includes immediate complications such as infections and bleeding, as well as long-term effects on fertility and the patient's psychological health.

- **Ethical considerations**: Students should also address the ethical implications of this surgery, particularly with regard to informed consent and the impact on the patient's quality of life after the procedure.

- **Case studies**: To enrich their understanding, it would be beneficial to include real-life case studies where orchiectomy has been performed, analyzing the patient's journey before and after the operation.

23. Practical work on erectile dysfunction and its treatment

Introduction

Erectile dysfunction, also known as ED, is a common problem affecting a significant proportion of men worldwide. This practical work aims to explore the causes, consequences and treatments available for erectile dysfunction. Students will be encouraged to examine these aspects from a variety of angles, including medical, psychological and social.

Practical work objectives

- **Understanding Erectile Dysfunction**: Define what erectile dysfunction is and identify its clinical manifestations.
- **Exploring the Causes**: Analyze the various causes of ED, including physical (cardiovascular disease, diabetes, etc.) and psychological (anxiety, depression) factors.
- **Examine the Consequences**: Discuss the emotional and relational impacts that ED can have on individuals and their partners.
- **Investigate Treatment Options**: Evaluate the different therapeutic approaches available, including..:
    - Oral medications (phosphodiesterase type 5 inhibitors)
    - Hormonal therapies
    - Mechanical devices (vacuum pumps)
    - Surgical procedures
    - Psychological therapies

Methodology: Students will be expected to carry out in-depth research into each aspect mentioned above. They may use case studies, academic articles and medical journals to support their analyses. Particular attention should be paid to statistical data concerning the prevalence of erectile dysfunction, as well as to the results of different treatments.

Presentation of results: Students must present their results in the form of a structured written report including:

- An introduction to the subject,
- A literature review on causes and consequences,
- A critical analysis of treatment options,
- Recommendations based on their research.

Conclusion

This practical work will enable students to gain an in-depth understanding of erectile dysfunction as well as academic research skills. They will also be encouraged to reflect on the social and personal implications associated with this condition.

24. Practical Work on Laparoscopic Inguinal Hernia Intervention

Laparoscopic inguinal hernia surgery is an increasingly common procedure that offers several advantages over traditional open surgery. This practical work aims to familiarize students with the principles, technique and post-operative considerations associated with this procedure.

Practical work objectives

- **Understanding of Theoretical Concepts**: Students should acquire a thorough knowledge of inguinal hernias, including their etiology, pathophysiology and surgical indications for treatment.

- **Learning Surgical Techniques**: Students will become familiar with the steps involved in laparoscopic surgery for inguinal hernia repair, including the use of specific instruments and anesthesia techniques.

- **Analysis of Advantages and Disadvantages**: A discussion of advantages (such as faster recovery and less post-operative pain) and disadvantages (potential risks such as nerve damage or anesthesia-related complications) should be included.

- **Hands-on simulation**: Students will take part in a simulated procedure, using anatomical models or surgical simulators to practice instrument handling and suturing.

- **Post-Operative Assessment**: Students will learn to assess a patient after a laparoscopic procedure, identifying signs of potential complications such as infection or bleeding.

Detailed content of practical work

1. Introduction to Inguinal Hernias: Inguinal hernias are defined as the displacement of an organ or tissue through a weak point in the abdominal wall. They can be classified into direct and indirect hernias, each with its own clinical characteristics.

2. Indications for surgery: Surgery is generally indicated when the hernia causes pain, discomfort or risk of strangulation. The surgical decision should be based on a thorough clinical assessment.

3. Surgical technique: Laparoscopic repair involves several key steps:

- **General anesthesia**: The patient is placed under general anesthesia.
- **Abdominal insufflation**: A gas (usually carbon dioxide) is insufflated into the abdominal cavity to create a working space.
- **Trocar insertion**: Trochars are inserted to provide access for surgical instruments.
- **Hernia repair**: The hernia sac is reduced and a prosthetic mesh is placed to reinforce the inguinal floor.
- **Closure**: Incisions are closed with sutures or staples.

4. Potential complications: Complications may include :

- Infection
- Hematoma
- Persistent pain

- Recurrence of hernia

5. Post-operative follow-up: Post-operative follow-up is crucial to monitor the patient's vital signs, manage pain and ensure there are no complications.

Conclusion

This practical work will enable students to acquire not only a theoretical but also a practical understanding of laparoscopic procedures to treat inguinal hernias, thus enhancing their future surgical skills.

25. Practical work on what to do in the event of genital ulceration

Introduction

Genital ulceration is a clinical symptom that can result from a variety of etiologies, from sexually transmitted infections (STIs) to dermatological diseases. It is crucial for medical and healthcare students to learn how to assess and manage these ulcerations appropriately. This practical work aims to provide a framework for the assessment, differential diagnosis, and management of genital ulcerations.

Practical work objectives

- **Understanding Etiologies**: Identify possible causes of genital ulcerations, including viral infections (such as herpes), bacterial infections (such as syphilis), and other dermatological conditions.
- **Clinical assessment**: Learn how to take a complete history and perform a targeted physical examination.
- **Differential diagnosis**: Draw up a list of potential diagnoses based on the clinical features of the ulcerations.
- **Management**: Discuss treatment options, including preventive measures and patient education.

Stages of practical work

- **Anamnesis**
    - Gather information on the patient's medical history, including previous STIs, associated symptoms (pain, itching), and sexual history.
    - Ask questions about the appearance of lesions: date of onset, evolution, precise location.
- **Physical examination**
    - Perform a complete physical examination, paying particular attention to the genital area.
    - Note the size, shape, number and appearance of ulcerations (purulent exudate, crusts).
- **Differential diagnosis**: Draw up a list of possible diagnoses:
        - Genital herpes
        - Syphilis
        - Soft canker
        - Lichen planus
        - Autoimmune diseases
- **Diagnostic tests**: Discuss appropriate diagnostic tests such as :
        - Viral culture or PCR for herpes virus.
        - Serological tests for syphilis (Wassermann test).
        - Skin biopsy if necessary.
- **Management**: Present the treatment options according to the established diagnosis:
        - Antivirals for herpes.
        - Antibiotics for bacterial infections.
    - Importance of patient education on STI prevention.

- **Ethical and psychological discussion**
    - Address the psychological implications of an STI diagnosis.
    - Discuss confidentiality and informed consent in the context of treatment.

Conclusion

This practical work will enable students to gain a thorough understanding of genital ulceration, as well as practical skills essential for their future medical careers.

26. Practical work on Trichomonas vaginalis

Introduction to Trichomonas vaginalis

Trichomonas vaginalis is a flagellate protozoan responsible for trichomoniasis, a common sexually transmitted infection (STI). This single-celled parasite primarily infects the urogenital tract of humans, causing a variety of symptoms and complications. Understanding this microorganism is essential for students of biology, medicine and public health.

Practical work objectives

- **Morphological identification**: Students will observe samples of T. vaginalis under a microscope to identify its morphological features, such as its pyriform shape, flagella and nucleus.

- **Parasite culture**: Students will learn to culture T. vaginalis from clinical specimens using appropriate culture media such as Diamond medium or TPY (Trypticase Peptone Yeast Extract) medium.

- **Analysis of Clinical Symptoms**: Students will study the symptoms associated with T. vaginalis infection in men and women, including vaginitis, urethritis and other clinical manifestations.

- **Diagnostic methods**: Students will explore different diagnostic methods for detecting T. vaginalis, including direct microscopic examination, culture and molecular tests such as PCR (polymerase chain reaction).
- **Treatment and Prevention**: A section will be devoted to the treatment options available for T. vaginalis infection, as well as prevention strategies to reduce transmission.
- **Ethical discussion**: Students will be invited to reflect on the ethical implications of STI testing and treatment, taking into account the associated social stigma.

Conclusion

This practical work aims to provide students with a thorough understanding of Trichomonas vaginalis, both microbiologically and clinically. By combining theory and practice, they will acquire essential skills in public health and microbiology.

Appendix 2: Bibliography

1. The Healing Power of Illness: Understanding the Mind-Body Connection" by Dr. Edward Bach
2. Mind Before Medicine: Scientific Proof That You Can Heal Yourself" by Dr. Lissa Rankin
3. The body remembers: the psychophysiology of trauma and its treatment" by Babette Rothschild.
4. "The Tao of Healing: a practical guide to traditional Chinese medicine" by Dr. Stephen T. Chang
5. "Anatomy of a disease: as perceived by the patient" by Norman Cousins
6. "Surgery: A Historical and Contemporary Perspective" by Sir Fredderick Treves
7. "The Principles and Practice of Surgery" by Sir William Osler
8. "Introduction to the study of surgery" by John Hunter
9. "Anatomy and surgical techniques: a pocket manual for the surgeon" by Dr. Joseph Lister
10. "The Surgical Clinics of North America" (edited by Dr. Charles H. Mayo)
11. "On Becoming a Person: Therapiest's View of Psychotherapy" by Carl Rogers
12. "The Interpretation of Dreams" by Sigmud Freud
13. "Man's Search for Meaning" by Viktor E. Frankl
14. "The Art of Loving" by Erich Fromm
15. "Healing the Shame That Binds You" by John Bradshaw

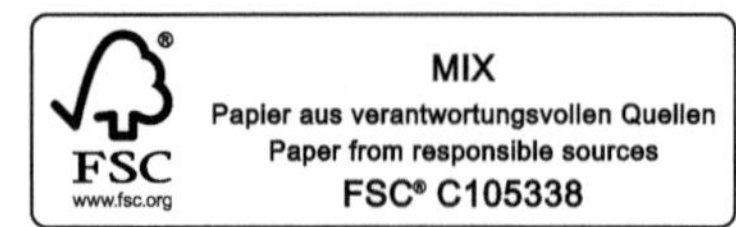

Printed by Books on Demand GmbH, Norderstedt / Germany